Successful Sleep Strategies from Birth to 3 Years

By

Sofia Hashemi

Table of Contents

In this section.

Treating a newborn who shouts non-stop? Who's a 1-year-old teething? A night terror preschooler?

In this section, you may learn how to deal with these problems and many more, while outlining the best sleep methods for every child's age and stage. In Section 4 you learn why your baby so frequently wakes you up with facts about the colic (and why this is not so frightening more) and critical information about SIDS prevention. Section 5 discusses sleep six months to a year and how you may benefit from a great opportunity: the new capacity for your kid to comprehend the pattern.

Section 6 explains what sleep patterns occur as your infant begins to stand and walk and why worry with separation may entail nights without bed. In Section 7 you may learn what to anticipate from the sleep when your child begins to speak and we offer you advice on how to deal with nightmares, night terrors and sleep wandering. You also find out how to manage this great transition in life: moving from the cot to a grown-up bed. And Section 8 deals with two main events of life, pre-school and toilet, affecting both daytime sleep and night sleep.

Section 4

Sleep from birth till 6 months Change and growth:

In the Section

- Take a look at the new sleep habits of your infant
- Plans for night-long sleep
- To protect your baby from SIDS
- Colic decontamination

Congratulations! As a brand-new parent, after so many hard months, you have one of our happiest experiences: holding your beautiful baby son or daughter in arms. Nothing can prepare you for the combination of love and amazement when you gaze at that tiny face and realize what an incredible donation you have had.

You will have to spend most of these early months walking clouds if you are like most new parents. Naturally, no matter how happy you are, you are like a zombie, understanding that sleeping for a decent night has been a luxury of the past (at least for now).

Whatever state you may be, happy or zombified — or both! — remember one word throughout the first six months: changing.

We explain in this Section the significant changes that occur throughout the first six months of your child's life and the relationship between sleep and your child. You also learn why some children believe that daytime is to sleep and evening is to party — a pattern that already stressed parents may tear out their hair. (It isn't only transitory, don't worry!) Moreover, you receive the inside history of treatments for colic, the advantages and disadvantages of pacifiers, and the key measures to keep you young.

The Early Development of

Babies

In the last six months of life, no other moment is as changing as a newborn.

During some spurts, the weight gain rate is 50 pounds per year, and the growth rate is 24 pounds per year. (Happily, it is just temporary otherwise you would need a larger crib!)

Your young child quickly acquires new skills and interests with that astounding physical development. She doesn't know how to speak, move from one place or envision anything beyond today. Yet she takes her first steps in one year, testing sounds or even words and develops an active, aware imagination.

During that period, she develops from complete dependency to a wonderful little person with a flourishing intellect and her own personality.

As the first several months pass, something else changes: the capacity to sleep of your kid. It comes out a little better every week, and slowly but surely, she does. This weird affair of snoring and waking a little better.

Two months' time:

Sweetheart meets world

It's wonderful how long a baby has been sleeping — and how frequently he rouses you out of bed at the same time. Consider his waking life in order to understand how his infant sleeps and why he must wake up so frequently.

The novelty of everything: Imagine going to the vast, light, brilliant, chaotic world from the warm, cosy womb predictability.

The changes that growing ups experience, such as relocating to a new city or changing professions, seem little in contrast.

The whole routine absence: The baby has no idea what will happen in two, two hours or even two minutes during the following two days. Such Hell may surprise even his own poops! The world is totally fresh and unexpected from his point of view.

What time it is, knowing it: Baby meets rhythm circadian

Many little animals know what to do from the start of their existence. Fish begin to swim; spiders begin to spin. However, human infants have no clue what to do next since they have

Greet the world considerably early than most other animals in its growth. Have you been born with an inherent personality and the color of father's hair or dimple, but a feel for everyday work?

They are clueless.

This absence of programming makes your kid incredibly flexible — he may fall into almost any pattern of life — and one of life's greatest wonders is the thrilling possibility to accomplish anything and to become a person. But fresh life begins with disadvantages when it comes to everyday activities.

The other side of your baby's ability for adaptation is that he's got a biological clock to begin with from scratch. Thus, the little time-speaking molecules in his body only guess wildly about day and night — which means that at any moment of the day or evening he may feel famished, tired and fully awake.

About one third of infants come to right, another third is at the ballpark and one third is off-base (so it's definitely good to have a baby with a proper internal alarm clock). As a consequence, the greatest difficulty during the first six months is that of most new mothers and fathers.

But even children have their own day/night cycle sensing rhythm. Like all people, infants have a circadian rhythm – a strong inner clock that helps build an everyday cycle. (For specifics, see Section 2.) At about 6 weeks old most of the kids feel weary throughout the night, become aware at daytime, feel hungry during hours of daylight rather than after darkness, and even prefer to snuggle a little more in the evening. They begin to understand that the day is for play, exploration and food, but it's time for night to take it easy.

A very powerful day and night reversal develops one three-third of infants who receive this cycle reversed. In the middle of the night, they are so hungry, they cannot be awakened by a storm during the day. This is excellent proof, albeit it is set in the wrong time zone, of the power of circadian rhythms!

Recognizing The major surprise of Baby: The feeling of starvation

Your tiny dumpling spent almost its entire existence sleeping in his first six months in the womb. He snoozed nearly continuously even in the third trimester. It was just a ticket to sleep all day and night.

So why is he not sleeping right now? Good question. - Good question. Mum's body provided all the nourishment he required before he arrived on the outer world.

But he wakes up in his stomach with this particular feeling — famine. He doesn't know, but he knows intuitively what to do —

weep! This is his only method to communicate "feed me." This is his only way.

Cribs stories: three methods, three successful families

At the age of 5 months, every four- or five-hours tiny Keiko woke up. Keiko began to sleep entirely on her own throughout the night in the middle of her fifth month — and she has done so ever since.

On the other hand, Molly and Jack felt urgent to sleep all night long. When Billy was four months old, Molly and Jack began utilizing Section 5 techniques to assist him find out how to sleep through the night.

Laura, the eldest of three children, saw her mother plucking her siblings in her crib, shutting the door and waiting for them to rest. She understood that method was working quickly and she attempted it with her child Sarah. At the third night, Sarah was only whispering. By the fourth, practically before Laura shut the door, she was sleeping.

What was the correct decision for the parents? They all—
because they have chosen the finest options for their lives and
kids.

And kid, he's gotta eat! Astonishing food is needed to
encourage the fast development of newborns. When you
compute its calorie consumption per pound, your intake will be
5-fold. Your young one is like a lumberjack wolfing food down
and he can't just do it or burst.

He is using a clever strategy: he sucks as much as his stomach is
able to keep him down then drifts asleep for two or three hours
again to sleep (three to four if you're fortunate) until his tummy
tells him again. Then for more he hollers. For at least the first
few weeks, he has to eat this frequently around the clock. And
during the first two months, your greatest strategy? Total
abandonment.

At this point, your baby has an airtight reason to take you out of
bed every couple of hours. Then for the first two months let him
call the shots. This is to feed him each time he shouts and
surrender himself to sleep. Go for a long, luxury sleeping
goodbye. Seek to catnap for a few hours while your infant
sleeps and be pleased with the opportunity.

In all this turmoil there is a luminous side: As you wait for this
child's hand and foot, astonishing pleasure comes to you in
taking care of this little person. Your own routine impacts are
changing completely

At the age of 5 months, every four or five hours tiny Keiko woke
up. Keiko began to sleep entirely on her own throughout the

night in the middle of her fifth month — and she has done so ever since.

On the other hand, Molly and Jack felt urgent to sleep all night long. When Billy was four months old, Molly and Jack began utilizing Section 5 techniques to assist him find out how to sleep through the night.

Laura, the eldest of three children, saw her mother plucking her siblings in her crib, shutting the door and waiting for them to rest. She understood that method was working quickly and she attempted it with her child Sarah. At the third night, Sarah was only whispering. By the fourth, practically before Laura shut the door, she was sleeping.

What was the correct decision for the parents? They all— because they have chosen the finest options for their lives and kids.

Your system will concentrate on your cherub completely and passionately.

You have to physically take care of who he is, what he wants and whenever he wishes. This all-round, albeit stressful, connection sometimes brings you closer to your little one, maybe as near as you can, if you're short on shuteye.

A gleam of hope to catch:

Two to four months

One night something amazing is happening while your kid is 6-16 weeks old: You will wake up, wake up, glance at your clock, and think, "Wow! Six whole hours I was sleeping!" Naturally, the very reason that you are surprised is because these frequent foods are not yet a past.

However, this magical moment is a great lot as it is the first step of your infant towards civilization. She is in the groove — she fits her environment — and she does it all by herself.

Your child's life has until now been a whirl of unexpected and frequent sleep breaks throughout the day and night. But all of a sudden, your baby stays awake throughout the day for extended periods. She starts to grasp the essential aspect of being human without the planning, preparation or charts (without even reading this book!)—the capacity to remain up long enough to study, work and spend. For a great deal of the day, she is very awake and alert — and you really feel like a light for much of the night.

In addition, less chaos:

Four to six months

When they reach the 4-month mark (donate or take a few weeks), almost every baby teases their relatives with a surprise night. However, these smart kids have a secret, which they do not typically disclose: most of them can now sleep without a meal or a visit from mom or daddy.

Some infants leave their parents in stealth and sleep all by themselves during the night. Three, seven and eventually nine hours of continuous slumber are spanned by these tiny ones. If you don't have it in your home, look for answers to your nighttime problems in the following part, "Guidance your baby on the way to mature sleep."

Guiding the way to mature sleep for your baby

You probably feel a bit confused right now if you are like many parents. Firstly, you want to sleep like an ordinary person again. On the other hand, you may think, "My child grows up too quickly, since you realize that your child is ready to sleep all night — his first major step into a gigantic universe.

And thus, you may have mixed emotions about his night's sleep without a food or hug around the 4-month mark.

But as he begins to sleep overnight, you have plenty of time for embraces and cuddling throughout the day.

Moreover, for fun, you have a lot more energy. So take it to heart and don't be afraid of this move forward - pleasure is only the start!

Set the inner clock for your baby

As we discussed previously in this Section, many infants require assistance to fit their circadian rhythm—and who can help better than their beloved parents? The joyous news is that even young owls ultimately become quite regularly awake at daytime and sleep at night, and this transition normally takes just six to eight weeks. This change does not take longer. These lengthy weeks however, by allowing Mother Nature's signals loud and clear, you may assist your baby reset the tiny clock faster. This is how:

Then open the windows and let the light to flow in throughout the day. Play music, create a lot of business and activity while the weather is good, and plan a little outside excursion.

Just the other way round when darkness comes. Turn the lights down, create as little noise as possible, turn the TV and radio off. Avoid chatting, too, for the most part. (In the Goodnight Moon even this "silent elderly woman saying hush" must have her lips scrubbed!) Feed, hug, massage, and as silently as possible cradle your baby.

These easy methods assist eliminate distraction and enable the body of your kid to take care of the last clock sets, local sunrise and sunset. In time, the rhythm of the Sun may lead to chemical processes, resetting the inner clock of your kid. And that is why flip flops become a spirit of the past, day and night – at least till adolescent years!

Home on the bandit of

sleep: You

You may be encouraged by news that your condition is transitory when you stand up every day of the night when your kid reaches its 4-month mark. Most children are ready to sleep through the night at this age. You're astonished when you compare photos of your little, dry baby with the roly-poly bambino you have now – and they grow much more slowly. They've plumped beautifully. Your stomachs no longer have to full in the middle of the day, and most can comfortably sleep. Both skills – feeding and sleeping sufficiently – are all that a baby must accomplish during the night.

There is just one explanation for it, when your kid wakes up when he achieves certain milestones. Your infant is in and out of deep slumber while it sleeps (more on this in Section 2). When he reaches that almost awake moment, he's had to make a decision: wake up or go back to sleep? If he picks Door No. 1 it is because you always have a food and a cuddle from your bed.

You first need to make a choice to deal with this situation:

Are you hopeless to get through the dormant stage?

Would you want to wait a few more months to encourage your child to quit his midnight demands?

Whether option is all right, you have to determine what works best for your lifestyle, job schedule and cleanliness. If you feel fully ready to proceed with helping your infant sleep all night, Section 5 walks you through the steps. Otherwise, the following part helps you weigh and decide on your choices.

I know when you are ready to abandon the snuggles at night

Just as your 4-month infant comes out of the newborn period in the anticipation of a 24-hour call, you, too, have gained certain expectations – the most important thing to hustle when your child shouts. In this way, each one of you has a pattern. "Wake up, weep, wait till mom or dad shows up," he says. "Wake up, listen and answer," is yours.

A few months ago, the call-and-response mode made great sense, but now both you and Baby are familiar with it. Now you may change your habit or you can wait as long as you like. Three methods (there is no right or wrong choice here) of approaching this phase are:

When she calls for you may continue to go to your kid. You'll be weary for a few more weeks, but at this point in time you can't pamper your kid or make permanent patterns. You may choose your child to sleep all night if you are fortunate. You're going to be off of the hook if so.

If you're confident she's alright, you may just stop answering your child's screams. You may anticipate your kid to scream for two nights bloody kills and then go to sleep angels. This is the fastest way to sleep through the night, but also one a lot of parents can't handle. That is not a trauma to your kid, but don't attempt it if it makes you uncomfortable.

You may use our Section 5 methods to easily but steadily make your infant sleep pattern entire night. These methods work for almost every baby over four months of age. (Although infants are usually prepared for this 4-month strategy, many parents are not!)

No matter whatever choice you choose, you must abide by one essential rule: Don't midstream change your mind! Weigh your choices, choose your best, and then stay for at least one or two weeks, to offer your child the greatest opportunity to adjust. Otherwise, you're confusing your child and she's spending many evenings trying out which game you're playing. It's much simpler for you both to adhere to your firearms.

Security First, but

Comfort too

Regardless of your sleeping technique, two things are important: safeguard your angel and make him comfortable.

Here are our highlights in both directions.

Keep your child secure throughout sleep.

No subject is more essential in terms of infants and sleep than safety — and no safety issue for kids under 1 is more vital than sudden infant death syndrome (SIDS). See the latest SIDS Statement at http://pediatrics. aappublications.org/cgi/reprint/116/5/1245 of the American Academy of Pediatrics for an outstanding overview of this topic. A overview of SIDS and how to keep your total safe. This part.

Understand what SIDS means

SIDS is one of the worst tragedies of life. Luckily this is uncommon and becoming more infrequent. More than 1 in 1,000 babies suffered from SIDS in 1991. This rate decreased by 50 percent by 2001 thanks to improved security measures; SIDS currently affects just over 1 in 2,000 infants. Almost 1,999 of every 2,000 infants do not fall prey to SIDS to put these numbers in perspective for the worn parents.

The term "SIDS" is used by the doctors to characterize any unexpected and inexplicable death in the first infant year. Most SIDS occurrences (about 75%) occur in the 1-4 months of age, with risk decreasing quickly after this time. In preterm kids and newborns exposed to cigarette smoke, AIDS occurs more often (though still seldom).

The danger increases with preterm newborns' severity (see Section 12 for details about prematurity). SIDS risk is approximately twice that for fully-term newborns, with increasing prematureness and closer to term for infants who are born 28-32 weeks of pregnancy. Certain research have shown that the risk of SIDS for a newborn exposed to smoking is five times greater (more in the next section).

For two causes, SIDS rates are declining:

SIDS is only explicit fatalities, by definition. With more medical issues that contribute to SIDS continued to be identified, less instances are unexplained.

Doctors revealed this magnificent finding a few years ago:

It may reduce the risk of SIDS by just half by placing a kid to sleep on the back rather than on her pum! By following this advice, parents reduce the danger.

Protect your child from SIDS

Recall: Back to Sleep if you remember nothing else, we teach you about nighttime safety. Just stated, always sleep your infant on his or her back. Note: No sleep on your side also. It isn't as dangerous as it's on its back, but it isn't as safe.

What if your kid turns his tummy from behind? The established notion is that mobile infants are at reduced risk for SIDS since they may move away from an uncomfortable or stressful situation. Don't be too worried if you see his kid on your back afterwards.

The back-to-back rule is one method to safeguard your child from the danger of SIDS. More recommendations may assist to keep the person secure are identified in the following list. (This list contains initially, but sure to read them all, the most potent methods.)

The danger factor to SIDS is extremely high to smoke. Some studies have shown that, when the infant is exposed to cigarette smoke during or after pregnancy, the risk of a baby is five times greater.

Be extremely cautious not to expose your child to cigarette smoke since this is one of the most significant risk factors for SIDS!

Do your best to stop when you are a smoker who reads this book before your baby comes. Have the whole house become a smoke-free zone if your child is already here. The risk of SIDS is increased even by second-hand smoking from one story away.

Some research indicate that there is a significant relationship between SIDS and soft bedding, pillows and face sheets. We don't know why, but even if your kid sleeps on his back, soft bedding is hazardous. If Baby has soft mattress, fluffy pillows or blankets that protect his face, the risk of SIDS may be up to five times higher.

Couches, sofas and waterbeds aren't ideal places to sleep.

All of them may raise the danger of SIDS, nixing it up and putting your candy on a genuine mattress bed.

SIDS risk may be decreased by pacifiers (see the "The pacifier power" section). However, numerous studies show that using a pacifier may decrease the risk of SIDS more than 50%. The degree to which it can minimize this risk remains unclear.

The environment of the baby should be comfortable but not too hot (65 to 72 degrees F). This simple adjustment may decrease the risk of SIDS so that the thermostat is not cranking.

The risk of SIDS is reduced when breastfeeding is linked. However, studies connect this protection to the fact that women who are breastfeeding tend less to smoke. The incidence of SIDS seems less in breastfeeding babies. Special protection against SIDS does not seem to be provided by breastfeeding itself. Don't worry about increasing the risk of SIDS if you feed your kid bottle. (Breastfeeding provides, of course, a lot of additional health benefits.)

While this is a contentious topic, sleeping together may raise the risk of SIDS. In Section 9, we examine the issue of cobordance and whether the risk of SIDS rises or reduces. If you sleep together, please ensure that we read and obey the guidelines for bed safety (as well as the smoking and alcohol taboos) we mention here.

There is no evidence of work for gadgets and gimmicks. The proof is clear: Products claiming to prevent or decrease SIDS, including home monitors and even prescription units, have not shown useful or safe. (The monitors, however, have their role to safeguard preterm babies from another respiratory issue – see Section 12.)

The use of peacemaker's

power

You have many methods to do anything when you're boring or scary — send a buddy via email, take a bike trip, read a nice book, cuddle up on the sofa, watch a TV...

Your young one has a very brief range of amusement choices, on the other hand. She is too new to read a book, and the storyline of Days of Our Lives is even a bit above her head. It is too early to read a novel (thank you, goodness!). So, she's doing what she does best—sweating things.

Sucking is one of the top ten favorite hobbies for every infant (just right there with snuggling and looking at wallpaper patterns). Eating is one of the very few activities your baby has done soon after birth. In reality, it relies on feeding to its life, and therefore the desire to suck is strong. Many infants get frenzied if they have nothing to suck on for a very long time.

Enter the pacifier — with several major benefits:

It's a wonderful comfort to find out how to fall asleep for your infant.

It is safe (in fact, it may reduce your baby's risk of SIDS by sucking at a pacifier—see preceding section).

You can wash it easily.

Pacifiers, on the other hand, have a few disadvantages:

A few infants who use a pacifier may refuse to nurse. This often occurs during the first three weeks of a baby's nursing. When your infant has mastered breastfeeding, pacifiers are far less likely to create feeding difficulties.

Pacifiers are often misplaced in the middle of the night. However, the majority of parents believe that the odd squawk from a baby who has misplaced her binkie is a reasonable trade-off for the hours of quiet provided by a pacifier. Additionally, when you begin to use the sleep techniques outlined in this book, your baby develops the ability to console herself when her favorite piece of plastic disappears.

Pacifiers may cause teeth to move forward in a newborn. Fortunately, pacifiers damage just the baby teeth and not the adult teeth. Therefore, if you can wean your child off the pacifier before she reaches five years old — and we strongly advise you to do so! — her next set of teeth will come in just fine.

Another criticism is that they are difficult to stop. Generally, this is not true. If you decide to discontinue using the pacifier within the first year or two, it may be surprisingly simple to do so. If your toddler is older and has a working knowledge of language, discuss the adjustment with him or her in advance.

(One ploy: Whether your family is expanding, check if your toddler is willing to offer the pacifier to the new addition as a present.)

Pacifiers, in general, are a gift rather than a curse, since they spare you and your baby a lot of pain — particularly on those nights when your darling struggles to sleep. We believe they are an excellent option.

The Greatest Common Obstacle: Colic Myths and Facts

Inquire of a physician, "What is colic?" and you get the following response: "A condition of prolonged and intense weeping lasting more than three hours per day that has no known reason and does not react to normal comforts such as feeding, massages, being held, or having a diaper changed."

However, ask a parent and you're likely to hear, "It's a nightmare — an eternity of shrill cries capable of sanding an elephant's ears off; a form of torture that makes bamboo splints under the fingernails sound like child's play; a horrifying experience of listening to your baby suffer at decibel levels capable of shattering glass!"

Both definitions seem to be fairly straightforward, yet for years, this frequent and distressing issue was the subject of unusual debate. The key issue was: Is colic a genuine illness, or are infants who experience colic in agony as a result of a severe medical problem?

Until recently, physicians were left with little clues. They were aware:

Colic-affected infants usually exhibit no symptoms of distress at delivery.

They develop a variety of difficulties around the age of one month.

Around three months of age, they revert to normal.

Placing colicky infants on a vibrating surface often alleviates their discomfort.

Because these data were few, colic remained a mystery until the 1990s (and even a little afterwards).

The colic myths

Over the years, physicians have concocted many hypotheses regarding the origins of colic. They were all incorrect, but we're going to explain a few of them so you're prepared in case you're the victim of one.

The worst notion was that stressed parents produced colicky infants, which resulted in needless guilt for zillions of parents. Fortunately, this idea was discarded before you became a parent — but you may still hear it from a distant cousin.

Recently, physicians believed that a colicky infant had not matured enough to manage emotions. As a consequence, according to this hypothesis, infants who lacked the ability to control their emotions burst into bouts of weeping and couldn't stop. However, this hypothesis left an important issue unanswered: Why do colic infants seem to be in so much physical pain?

Colic facts

Recent medical discoveries have shown that the majority of instances of colic are caused by two simple (although unpleasant) conditions: allergies and stomach acid. This finding is very beneficial for parents since both issues have safe, quick, and easy solutions. Here's the lowdown on each offender and his or her remedy:

Allergies are the primary antagonist.

Previously, doctors believed that infants could not develop allergies until they reached the age of two. However, physicians have found that many infants who cry in agony have irritated intestines due to dietary allergies. When their parents stop feeding them the items to which they are allergic, these infants almost immediately recover from colic and resume regular bowel movements.

Additionally, the proteins in a mother's diet may flow directly into her breast milk unaltered. Therefore, if you consume yogurt for lunch and subsequently nurse a baby who is lactose intolerant, you may anticipate complications.

Combine these two facts — that little children may be allergic to certain meals and that even breastfeeding mothers can supply the foods that give them pain — and you have one very solid solution to the question, "What causes colic?"

If this is the case with your infant, work with your doctor to determine which foods trigger the response and then remove them:

If Mom is nursing, the bad guys are often proteins from cow's milk, soy, or other foods, and the solution is for Mom to discontinue all consumption of the problematic foods.

If Baby is bottle-fed, the soy or cow's milk in infant formulae may be the source of the issue; the remedy is to give your baby an elemental formula (all proteins have been broken down; the formula is still nutritious but does not cause allergies). Your doctor can advise you on the appropriateness of this strategy for your child.

Tummy acid is the villain number two.

For years, physicians overlooked stomach acid as a possible cause of colic for the same reason they overlooked allergies: they believed infants were too young to have this issue.

Recent studies, however, established the contrary. Heartburn (a.k.a. reflux or gastroesophageal reflux disease, GERD) may make infants as uncomfortable as it does adults.

Heartburn happens when stomach acid burns the lining of your esophagus or intestine (the sections immediately before or following the stomach). While the majority of individuals have stomach acid that is capable of creating this issue, they also have protective linings — similar to oven gloves — that prevent the acid from reaching sensitive areas. If a breach develops in the liner, the acid may seep through and burn... Ouch! However, you may wonder, since almost everyone gets stomach acid and nearly all infants have acid wash up into their esophagus (do you know any babies who never spit up?), why do only some babies have heartburn? We don't know — but we do know that a large number of infants suffer from this condition.

When adults have heartburn, they often go for an antacid. However, infants have just one method of communicating their pain – they scream their hearts out. Fortunately, if your baby's discomfort and tears are being caused by heartburn, the following remedies may help:

Your doctor may prescribe safe and uncomplicated medicines that effectively prevent stomach acid production.

Stomach acid seems to be of little value, and its elimination appears to be harmless – at least for a few months, until your sweetheart outgrows the danger of heartburn.

Maintain an upright position for your infant after a meal to minimize the risk of that searing stomach acid splashing up into his throat.

Elevate the head of your baby's crib slightly, which also aids in the retention of stomach acid.

If you are bottle-feeding your infant, you may thicken the formula by adding a little amount of rice cereal. Again, this contributes to the retention of acid in the stomach, where it belongs.

While the majority of infants with colic have curable issues, a minority do not. These babies will scream their little hearts out for the first several months, even after physicians have ruled out all possible causes. The reason is almost certainly explicable... but medical science must find it. The good news is that even in this case, the weeping fits often subside after three months. Therefore, hold on – there is a light at the end of the tunnel!

Section 5

Getting the Hang of It: Sleeping Between the Ages of 6 and 12 Months

Throughout This Section

- Making the decision to sleep through the night
- Promoting a restful night's sleep
- Facilitating the process: Lovies, naps, and the aforementioned setbacks

Are you the only parent at your child's playgroup who still wears sunglasses to conceal dark bags beneath the eyes? If this is the case, do not despair. Babies have a broad variety of personalities and sleep needs, and some just need more time and support to establish a sleep pattern.

This Section teaches you how to coax your little darling into following a routine: by establishing your own bedtime ritual, adjusting the menu at mealtimes to promote longer sleep, and gently and lovingly limiting the nocturnal demands she puts on you. All of these methods add up to more sleep for you and your child (as well as more active days).

Sleep patterns of your infant do not change overnight (pun intended); it takes days, if not weeks. However, with enough perseverance, you will eventually achieve the nirvana of sleeping until the alarm clock sounds. And, given enough time, this stretch becomes the norm rather than the exception.

Recognize When You and Your Baby Are Prepared to Sleep Through the Night

Sleeping through the night is a significant milestone on the path to independence, and the first true decision your child has in her early life is whether or not to sleep. Meanwhile, you'll get a parenting gold star for assisting her in taking the first baby step toward becoming a big child.

The question is, "Can my little child survive a whole night alone?" has no one-size-fits-all solution. However, most infants are physiologically prepared to sleep through the night by the time they reach the age of four months. (For additional information on this preparedness, see Section 4.) Permanence of objects may aid in sleeping through the night without asking for parents and develops around the age of 9 months — we explore this subject in more depth in Section 6.

So why are we discussing this problem in a Section on infants aged six to twelve months? That is an excellent question! This is the stage at which the majority of parents feel comfortable imposing certain restrictions on their children. While some parents may begin experimenting sooner (with good cause), the majority prefer to wait until the six-month mark before taking active efforts to alter sleep routines. The strategy is sound because it almost ensures that your angel will be prepared — and that you will have had enough midnight hugs.

Because each family is unique, consider both your baby's preparedness and your own needs and emotions when determining if the time is appropriate for your infant to take this significant step.

Knowing when Baby is scheduled to sleep through the night

How can you be certain that your sweetie is prepared to spend the night alone in that crib? To assist you in making that choice, consider the following:

Is your infant capable of falling asleep on his own? In other words, if you place him in his crib before he falls asleep completely, can he take the last step to the Land of Nod on his own?

If your baby falls asleep on his own and does not need his evening snacks but still wakes you up at 1 or 2 a.m., he is likely more interested in some face time with Mom or Dad than in a meal. He's ready to sleep through the night now that waking up every few hours have become a pleasure, not a necessity. (For additional information on needs vs wants, see Section 1.)

Is it possible for your kid to eat all the calories he needs during daytime hours? Yes, unless your infant came prematurely (see Section 12 for information on early-bird feeding requirements). Babies as young as four months are large enough — and their development is modest enough — to avoid a midnight snack. (For particular ideas on how to reduce midnight feedings, see the following section "Using Calorie Shifting to Reset Your Baby's Clock.")

Is your kid healthy and free of a chronic condition that may interfere with sleep? A health condition may exacerbate feeding and sleep problems, so discuss any health concerns with your doctor before assuming that the runway is free for all-night sleeping. (For more information on coping with sleep and health issues, see Section 13.)

At this age, some infants do have genuine nocturnal requirements.

Babies who were born prematurely, are sick, or can only consume a little amount at a single meal may still need night feedings. In these instances, the methods described in this Section are still beneficial — but you should wait a few weeks or months before attempting them.

This begs the following question: Are you up to the task?

Ascertaining if you are on target

If your infant has the ability and maturity to sleep through the night, half the fight is over. The other part of the equation is keeping your own heart in the game.

If you're like the majority of parents, you're caught between the guilt of not fulfilling your baby's every request and the need for a decent night's sleep to reclaim your humanity. Perhaps you're privately angry of giving up that late-night hug, but you're also becoming more grumpy, tired, and (admit it) resentful with each loud scream that pulls you out of bed.

These competing feelings may affect your choice to sleep all night. However, at this point, the ball is in your court, not your infant's. There is no such thing as a correct or incorrect choice; thus, you must strike a balance that works for both you and your toddler. The following are a few pointers to assist you along the way:

Contrast assisting your infant in falling asleep with allowing your baby to scream. While crying is a sideshow (and you may hear a lot of it in the coming weeks!), it is not the primary problem.

Rather than that, keep this idea in mind: Are you still putting your baby to sleep, or has your baby discovered how to sleep on her own? Your objective is to assist her in achieving independence in this critical life skill, so don't allow her tears distract you. If she successfully manipulates you into feeling guilty, both of you will have many sleepless nights ahead of you.

If you're making this choice with a partner, ensure that both of you are completely committed to this move. If one spouse is prepared and the other is not, you will be unable to maintain consistency, and your child will mimic the more hesitant parent. It is preferable to wait a few weeks (or even months) before implementing your sleepy-time tactics fully.

When the moment is perfect, do a brief reality check with these reminders before putting your goals into motion:

Recognize that sleeping through the night has varying meanings for various individuals. Sleeping through the night ideally implies that both you and your baby feel refreshed and prepared to face the day. For some families, this means ten hours of beautiful sleep for their infant, while others are quite content with a short 2 a.m. feeding or an early human alarm clock.

Be prepared for some aggravation. For instance, do not be shocked if your little angel sleeps peacefully through the night for weeks and suddenly begins screaming like a banshee at 2 a.m. A baby's sleep is often disrupted just before significant developmental surges, and many of these surges occur between the ages of six and twelve months.

Establishing a Routine for

Bedtime

At this stage of your baby's life, regularity is critical. (By this, we mean a timetable for day and night activities that is predictable.) At this age, your baby is ready to establish a reasonably regular schedule for feeding and sleeping. If he hasn't quite mastered the scheduling thing, have no fear - this section contains practical strategies for assisting your child in adjusting his schedule to yours.

A few simple tips to get

you started

By six months of age, your baby begins to connect regular rituals with bedtime. The purpose of these rituals is to gently transition her from the activity of the day to the calm of the evening, psychologically and physically preparing her for bed.

You'll develop your own nighty-night routines over time, but the following principles work effectively for many parents:

Establish a bedtime. This time period may be variable, but it should be generally constant. Babies' sleep requirements vary, and average bedtimes range from 7 p.m. to 9 p.m.

Naturally, your job schedule and personal preferences play a role in your choice.

Avoid the misconception that keeping your baby up until she is really tired would encourage her to sleep in. That strategy is seldom successful — and almost always results in a big tantrum when she is overtired.

Consider the day she's had and maintain some wiggle room. For example, if your kid just visited Chuck E. Cheese, she is most likely overstimulated (and perhaps still recovering from the trauma of being hugged by a big rat), so make the nighttime routine as peaceful and quiet as possible. On the other hand, if she spent the day relaxing inside, she may not be enough exhausted to sleep properly. If that is the case, try if you can include a little activity before beginning your sleep ritual.

Make an early start. Set the tone for bedtime 30 to 45 minutes before you want to put your baby to sleep.

This may be accomplished by turning out lights, playing quiet music, and switching off the television.

If your kid is a baby, feed her before to bedtime, stopping when she seems sleepy but not quite asleep. You may need to gently awaken her to ensure she does not fall asleep too soon.

As previously said, most of the effort in getting your baby to sleep through the night is spent teaching her how to sleep on her own — which is why you don't want to do the job for her.

Prepare for success by dressing appropriately. Change your infant into soft, comfortable pajamas that are free of frills, buttons, or tags that may pinch, bind, or irritate. One of the most frequent errors is to overheat the bedroom before night.

Babies have the same ability as adults to regulate their body temperatures, so put your baby in the same weight of clothes that you are comfortable wearing.

Reduce the brightness of the lights. Certain infants sleep well in the dark, while others like a little amount of light. If your child falls into the second group, consider investing in a dimmer switch and dimming the lights during crib time. After your infant has fallen asleep, turn off the light.

This phase gradually acclimates her to sleeping in a completely dark environment (which can help keep sleep schedules on track). If your baby becomes used to sleeping in a dark room throughout his or her toddler years, the issue is less likely to be a problem.

Activities that assist your infant in winding down

Adults like reading a book, watching a little television, snacking, or taking a leisurely stroll to unwind before sleep. These rituals communicate, "Ignore the stresses of the day; it's time to unwind." Because your infant is incapable of doing any of these activities on his own, you must offer some quiet amusement before to sleepy time.

Consider a tubby-time. A little trial and error is required here, as some infants find baths relaxing, while others get energized in the tub. If bathing your baby helps him relax, give him one before changing him into his pajamas. If baths cause him to become hyperactive, plan them earlier in the day.

Give your kid your enchantment. A gentle rubdown may assist in dissipating stress and is an excellent way to connect with your kid.

Apply a little amount of oil to your hands (ordinary olive oil or baby oil works well!) and give your child a gentle, soothing head-to-toe massage.

Take time to read an excellent book. Story time is one of the greatest nighttime activities; short, rhyming tales with a sing-song rhyme or rhythm are very calming. Apart from assisting your infant in winding down, tales are an excellent method to promote language development. Section 17 has a plethora of ideas.

Sing a little song. Babies, too, like singing, and a gentle song while rocking may calm even the most alert infant.

Beyond the yawns, lulling

Baby

When your infant is on the verge of falling asleep, make your move.

Place her in her cot and whisper softly, "Good night, I love you, see you tomorrow." (And silently hope that you will not see her again till dawn!)

Many infants like to sleep to the sound of soothing music.

Musical patterns are very appealing to the brain and may help cover household noises that may be disturbing your child's sleep (particularly if other children are around – siblings sometimes struggle to turn down the volume when a little child is attempting to sleep). If you play the same tunes each night, the music will also serve as a signal to your infant that sleep is near.

How to Reset Your Baby's Clock Using Calorie Shifting

One of the most effective methods for assisting your kid in sleeping through the night is to reset his stomach clock. The objective here is calorie shifting, or gradually reducing your baby's evening meal intake without causing him to get hungry.

Calorie shifting is effective because the human body retains information about when it has been eaten. As a consequence, individuals develop eating habits depending on their eating schedules. For example, individuals who eat supper regularly around 10 p.m. are usually not hungry at 6 p.m., and vice versa.

The same holds true for your infant. If you consistently feed him at 2 a.m., his stomach will shout, "Feed me!" at 2 a.m. each day. If you want to eliminate the nighttime bottle or nursing, you must adjust his internal schedule — which is really very simple.

Do not be concerned about starving your child when you utilize the calorie shifting method. (If Grandma claims you are, she is incorrect.) At any given age, the majority of infants consume about the same number of calories per 24 hours. If you eliminate the midnight snack, your infant will just consume more calories throughout the day.

In essence, the calorie-shifting phase described in the following paragraphs is the culmination of a process that began with the introduction of cereals, fruits, and vegetables to your baby's diet. This adjustment resulted in a significant shift in your baby's feeding habits toward the afternoon. To guarantee restful sleep, you'll want to fine-tune that balance even more.

If you are breastfeeding

If you're nursing, breastfeeding mothers may still decrease the number of nighttime feedings their infants need. When your infant awakens in the middle of the night,

Try rubbing her back or singing to her to see if you can lull her to sleep without feeding her.

Determine which night feeding is of least interest to her and attempt to skip that one each night.

Send in Dad or another responsible adult to take care of the infant in place of Mom. Breast milk's fragrance may entice your infant to breastfeed.

If you're comfortable with bottles, try giving your infant a bottle of breast milk for night feedings, gradually diluting it until it's essentially water. (For further information, see the next section.) Again, fathers may have a better chance with this stage.

By this age, nipple confusion is no longer a problem (difficulty returning to nursing after switching to a bottle).

If you are bottle-feeding

you may promote calorie shifting by using the following dilution strategy:

Select the first night feeding to eliminate and make the formula for that meal 78% or 34% strength.

If your baby tolerates this bottle well and is content, gradually reduce the intensity of the formula by 1/8 or 1/4 until the bottle contains just water.

Rep this procedure for each nightly feeding; soon, your infant will be completely satisfied throughout the night. At this point, he's waking you up just for the purpose of having fun!

This is the time to softly and kindly alter the game's rules.

With Love, Establishing

Limits

When you're certain that your infant is receiving enough calories throughout the day, you may be quite certain that her main purpose for waking is to see you. This is a strong yearning that your infant anticipates being fulfilled.

The critical point, though, is that it is a want, not a need. Much of your time as a parent will be spent assisting your kid in distinguishing between desire and need, and the bedtime problem will serve as your first major test.

(Believe it or not, it's also one of the most straightforward.) Wait till you explain to your 13-year-old that she does not need makeup or your 16-year-old that he does not need his own vehicle!)

Begin by altering your child's habits

Changing this appear-on-demand habit begins with you, not your kid. Your first step is to recognize that if you alter the pattern, your kid will be OK. When you calmly and compassionately allow him to adjust to new expectations, you do not traumatize him at all (if you have any doubts, read our discussion of disappointment vs trauma in Section 1). The more authority you offer your child in discovering his or her ability to solve issues, the more confidence he or she develops in his or her own skills and abilities.

Of course, you are naturally predisposed to respond to those piteous shrieks, and therefore must see this circumstance as an opportunity for your angel to grow. You are not being harsh; you are being prudent.

Consider methods to

assist you on your journey

Now that you understand why your kid needs to sleep alone, it's time to get specific. Here's an excellent method for handing over the keys to Sleepy land to your love-bug:

When you hear your baby cry, pause for a moment or two. Each night, she'll cycle between deep and light sleep phases three to four times and may briefly awaken. If you rush to her at the first indication of awakening, she will not have time to naturally transition back to deep slumber.

Bear in mind that sobbing is not a pick-up line. If your child's scream sounds normal and you are certain she is OK, refrain from scooping her up. This may be a cue for play or perhaps a feeding. Rather than that, wait a few moments and let her to find her own way back to sleep.

If you're ready to make the switch to all-night sleeping, keep this slogan in mind: If at first you fail, try again... and again... and again! The ideal strategy is to establish a bedtime and wake-up time for your kid and to avoid entering his or her room in between — and consistency is the most important factor in success. If she even sees you once

Throughout this time period, you reinforce her perception that you present when she weeps. Typically, it takes between two and four nights for your kid to adjust her expectations, stop screaming, and sleep through the night.

Safety valves for use during periods of high pressure

Even in the best of circumstances, regulations must be bent somewhat. Here are a few suggestions:

Recognize when your infant is serious. If your darling is fully awake and his scream is unusually howling, a visit is in order. Ascertain that he is not ill, trapped, or soaking wet. If everything is OK, reintroduce him to his cot, massage his back, and communicate your presence to him in a soothing voice. While some infants need Mom or Dad to remain with them until they fall asleep, others settle down quickly and may be left alone while still awake.

Reintroduce reinforcements. We discussed previously in the section "If you're nursing" how the smell of breast milk may stimulate your baby's hunger. Obviously, this is not an issue if a man takes over the night shift! For these and other reasons — including those deep, rumbling masculine voices — males seem to have an advantage when it comes to coaxing infants to sleep. However, any replacement may assist, so ask a nanny, a mature adolescent, or a grandmother to take over night duties if you're fortunate enough to have one available at 2 a.m.

Don't berate yourself if your firmness isn't as strong as you'd want it to be. This may seem to contradict the consistency-is-critical guideline, but being at the beck and call of your darling little tyrant is a difficult habit to break. Picking up your child sometimes does not create a significant setback — but resist the temptation.

Taking Care of Logistical

Issues

Numerous variables, both big and little, contribute to the effectiveness of a sleep regimen. We'll look at three of them in this section: safety, comfort, and those all-important naps.

Assuring that your nursery is secure against an escape artist

The safety of your infant as she sleeps is paramount. To feel secure about creating a routine, you must first ensure that your baby's cot is really safe - even when she is alone.

Safety-proofing your baby's bedroom was simple in the early months. The regulations, however, are shifting now that your kid is moving in all directions – even up!

When your infant begins to pull himself up to a standing position:

- Remove bumper pads to prevent her from climbing up and falling out of the crib.
- Eliminate all low-hanging mobiles.
- Ascertain that she cannot reach curtain pulls, wall-mounted photos, or other possible hazards.
- Double-check the crib hardware to ensure it is secure.
- Ensure that all electrical outlets have safety plugs, even if you believe they are out of reach of your infant.
- You're going to be surprised at what she can get herself into and climb up to in the months ahead.
- Taking care of blankies and other heirlooms

As your baby enters the second part of his first year, you'll likely find that he develops an attachment to specific things — a cloth diaper, receiving blanket, or soft doll. If you ask your mother or father about their own babyhood, you're likely to learn that you, too, had a lovie that soothed you and made you feel secure.

These things are referred to be transitional artifacts because they serve as a reminder to youngsters of their parents' love and care.

In essence, the cherished blankie or dolly serves as a conduit between Mommy and Daddy and the need to be with them.

After your kid reaches the 12-month mark and is old enough to sleep with a plush toy or blanket, a lovie may be a huge aid at bedtime. When a kid awakens in the night, he or she may hug his or her particular lovie and use it to remember Mom or Dad's presence and be soothed back to sleep. Note: Do not be concerned if your kid lacks a favorite blanket or doll. Many infants do not, and they sleep well.

Rub your baby's lovie against your skin before placing it in the crib. This may seem disgusting, but putting a little amount of *eau-de-you* on the lovie may make it more reassuring at night.

Parents often have a love-hate connection with a certain lovie, the pacifier. Babies who fall asleep sucking on one may be perplexed when they cannot find it in the middle of the night; naturally, they cry for assistance — a particularly troublesome issue between the ages of four and eight months. (Subsequently, they seem to use baby sonar and locate the concealed reward on their own.)

To prevent the pacifier search in the middle of the night, try exchanging it for another lovie, such as a doll or blanket, and see whether your baby accepts the swap. Bear in mind, however, that new research indicates that pacifiers may help prevent against sudden infant death syndrome (SIDS). (See Section 4 for more information on pacifiers in general and SIDS prevention in specifically.)

An observation about

naps at this age

A sleep for a tired parent is like to a life preserver for a drowning person. Babies' naps offer parents with the necessary time to unwind and rejuvenate — and, of course, to read excellent parenting books. Naps are usually taken in the middle of the morning or afternoon.

Typically, children between the ages of 6 and 12 months sleep 10 to 12 hours at night and take two naps of approximately an hour each.

(Toward the end of the year, naps may be reduced to just one.) Naturally, it is the average amount of sleep – and as we all know, no kid is average! In fact, sleep requirements vary widely, and you have little influence over the overall number of hours your infant requires in a 24-hour period.

The good news is that you can utilize the same sleep techniques that you use at night (check the earlier sections of this Section for a review of these strategies). The key is consistency. Additionally, the following techniques may help encourage a pleasant naptime:

Timing: Maintain as much consistency as possible with your routine, but you do not need to drag your life to a grinding stop in order to put your baby down at the exact same times each day.

Consider the following suggestions:

• Schedule a half-hour nap after lunch or a snack to ensure that your baby's stomach is full; this will aid in her sleeping more peacefully.

• Adjust naptime if you feel your baby is becoming sleepy ahead of schedule. Otherwise, she is likely to get overtired and unable to sleep.

• Schedule your baby's second nap during the early afternoon to provide her enough time to fall asleep before night.

Sounds: Maintain a low level of noise in your home during naptime and play some quiet music in the background.

Consider purchasing blackout shades for the nursery, since small infants sleep better in a dark environment.

Toys: Once your child hits the 12-month milestone and crib toys are no longer considered inappropriate, put some safe toys in the crib. They can buy you a few priceless moments of peace and quiet by entertaining your baby when she opens her eyes for the first time.

Whatever you do to make naptime more appealing, be prepared for an occasional battle. At night, you have the upper hand because biology compels your infant to sleep — even if it seems to take an eternity. At naptime, your baby, on the other hand, has an ace up her sleeve: she is physically capable of refusing to sleep. To her, the world is so enticing that she may very well insist on being awake, regardless of how grumpy she becomes.

However, you are not required to fully surrender. Even if you are unable to induce sleep in your baby, you may put her in her cot and keep her there. She may protest the first few times you do this, but she ultimately gets the message — and grants you an hour or two of much-needed independence.

Recognizing and Combating Difficulties incurred as a result of Milestones

Milestones in your baby's development may have a significant impact on his or her sleep. Consider each developmental surge as a massive tidal wave approaching from behind. As you feel the approaching water, you tighten up in preparation for the wave. When infants approach a significant milestone, they, too, feel the stress, which often spills over into the sleep cycle.

Sitting up, crawling, and pulling up to a standing position are perhaps the most frequent developmental milestones that alter sleep patterns. At times, a toddler becomes so enthused about a new ability that he cannot sleep. At other instances, a child acquires a new ability, such as sitting or standing up in his crib, but hasn't learned the fine art of going back down; he squawks for assistance, unable to figure out how to plop back down on his bed. (For more on how to assist a child who becomes trapped in this manner, read Section 6.)

You may find it fascinating to keep track of your child's sleep-wake cycle variations to see if interruptions occur prior to the development of a new ability. Of course, this charting will have no effect on your child's sleep, but your awareness of this transient shift may provide you peace. Sleep often returns to normal after your infant has mastered the new ability.

To keep track of your baby's sleep, just use the forms included in this book's appendix to track the number of hours your baby sleeps each night and nap. After that, search for patterns. For example, five restful nights followed by four cranky nights or three missed afternoon naps in a row may indicate a significant development, like as learning to sit up or crawl. Additionally, charting may assist you in identifying patterns and determining the effectiveness of your sleep methods.

Section 6

Baby on the Move: Sleeping between the Ages of 12 and 18 Months

In This Section, we'll discuss...

- ➢ How to transition into separation-anxiety state.
- ➢ Practicing your abilities in the face of nocturnal obstacles and setbacks
- ➢ Revision of safety regulations, naps, and calming items

Consider the sensation of mastering a new skill every few weeks. In the adult world, that's the equivalent of becoming an expert guitarist, an excellent golfer, and a gourmet chef in a matter of months. That is how life is today for your kid, who is rapidly acquiring incredible abilities. What an exciting moment for your child in his or her second year of life!

Crawling and walking are two of the most important abilities. Although there is some variety, most youngsters begin crawling around the age of 9 months and progress to walking around the one-year mark. These shifts result in significant psychological alterations that usually manifest themselves soon after the 12-month mark.

Crawling and walking are significant milestones in your child's development because they broaden his or her physical and mental horizons. However, they also have an effect on your child's daytime and nightly sleep. Thus, just when you thought you were safe at home, you may be confronted with the restless nights that plagued you throughout your baby's first few months.

Along with crawling, standing, and walking, a condition known as separation anxiety may wreak havoc on your child's sleep.

Fortunately, sleep difficulties at this time are usually transitory, but we teach you how to deal with them using a few tried-and-true methods in this Section. Additionally, we discuss standing in the crib, why it may be a challenge for a toddler, and how you can assist your baby in swiftly resolving the issue.

Gaining Independence: The Exciting — and Terrifying!

Along with the euphoric sensation your one-year-old receives when he begins to make major choices (which toys to grasp, which sights to investigate), his newfound independence comes with a downside: He knows he has the ability to leave you... and you have the ability to leave him. Until now, he has seen you as a permanent fixture, similar to the couch or coffee table. However, he now understands that — unlike the furniture — you may flee to new lands. It's frightening news at first, and he reacts to imminent separations by clinging to your leg like a suckerfish, crying like a baby, or even having full-fledged hissy fits.

Your kid's panicked reactions to your absences — what child psychologists refer to as separation anxiety — are a typical developmental stage. Indeed, it demonstrates that your child is acquiring these critical new skills:

➢ He distinguishes between known and unfamiliar individuals.
➢ He understands how vital you are in his life.
➢ He has the foresight to foresee the heartbreaking sensation of missing you when you are gone.

However, he is unable to comprehend those partings are transitory, and therefore views them as frightening, even at sleep.

Separation is such a lovely agony: Separation anxiety begins

Separation anxiety is unpredictable, yet it is a natural byproduct of object permanence, the awareness that you do not just disappear when you are out of sight. Object persistence generally occurs between the ages of 8 and 12 months, whereas separation anxiety occurs between the ages of 12 and 20 months. Separation anxiety gradually subsides as your kid realizes that you will return after each separation.

When separation anxiety takes over, your kid — even if she has always been a people person — may abruptly withdraw when introduced to strangers. A sitter's arrival (even a familiar one) is also likely to result in tears or tantrums. Additionally, since the boundary between friend and stranger remains somewhat blurred

Each kid responds differently to separation anxiety. Some children cannot bear to be apart from their parents, while others glide through this period with just occasional clinginess.

Children's reactions to partings are heavily influenced by their personalities. While shy infants are often the most affected, even the most carefree and outgoing children may surprise their parents by developing a severe case of separation anxiety. Significant life events, such as a relocation or the birth of a sibling, may also elicit an acute dread of being separated from Mom or Dad.

Recognize why separation anxiety impairs sleep

When separation anxiety concerns arise, sleep problems often accompany them, since sleep is a significant separation for your child. At this point, he can predict how he will feel when left alone in his crib, and he lets you know – loudly — that he is not looking forward to your departure.

With these bloodcurdling shrieks, he communicates that he is intensely connected to you and relies on you to keep him safe and secure. Recognizing your baby's deep attachment to you may give you the warm fuzzies. However, when you realize it's back... the weekly nighttime battle... that warm sensation soon transforms to heartburn.

Taking Control of the Night: Overcoming Common Sleep Issues

Your child's growth path may seem to be a little rough right now, as she is actually taking two steps forward and then collapsing on her bottom. Likewise, her psychological growth is parallel to her physical development. The more she comprehends, the more she considers even the most trivial things. Your toddler's distress may result in some sleepless nights and difficult choices for you as you adjust to her developing demands and wants.

Because you cannot escape these developmental growth spurts (and you do not want to!), this section discusses some methods for calming your child.

Relieving separation anxiety throughout the night

Routine is especially critical for youngsters who are learning the thrilling but sometimes frightening skill of separation from their parents, since regular routines help to alleviate their worries during this stressful period.

This implies that toddlers thrive on regularity, so if you didn't develop a schedule for your kid during the second part of his or her first year (see Section 5 for suggestions), now is a good time to do so.

While consistency is desirable, bedtime routines must also adapt to your child's development. This adaptability implies that the books you read, the songs you sing, and the pre-bedtime snack your kid enjoys will vary. However, if your overall pattern is well-established, the little adjustments you make will have no effect on the bedtime process.

When you see the first symptoms of separation anxiety, reassemble the components of your sleepy-time drill (we cover the fundamentals of the routine in Section 5). This part includes some new components and changes appropriate for your child's age.

Adhere to a script. Utilize your child's developing language abilities while preparing him for sleep or other transitional periods. Each night as sleep approaches, repeat the same phrases to your infant in short, clear sentences (imagine Jane conversing with Tarzan). For example, a few minutes before your scheduled bedtime, you may remark, "Look at the clock - it's nearly bedtime!" Your kid will comprehend a surprising amount of this message, and the repetition will reassure him.

Maintain a solitary bath. A warm bath is an excellent way to welcome the sandman at this age. However, if you have several children, avoid cramming everyone into the tub at the same time. Two or more children in a bathtub brimming with toys, suds, and water is hardly a relaxing situation for anybody! If it is difficult to squeeze separate baths into each night, allow the cleaner child to miss a day.

Cozy up with a good book. Even if you add new books as your kid grows older, return to the classics often — particularly during difficult periods such as the separation-anxiety phase.

Resist the temptation to fudge bedtime. While it may be tempting to keep a kid up a bit longer (particularly if Mommy or Daddy returns home late), this switch simply overstimulates your child and disturbs the nighttime routine.

Rather than that, consider scheduling family time for a few additional minutes in the morning, when everyone has slept well.

Allow Teddy to work the evening shift. Now that your darling has passed the one-year mark, he is legally allowed to sleep with a doll or stuffed animal (see the safety tips at the end of this Section). You may include this lovie into your night routine.

For example, invite Teddy to join you during story time and then tuck him up and say "Night-night" to him as well.

While the sun is still up, squelching separation anxiety

Stress from a busy day may lead anybody to toss and turn, and this is true for children as well as adults.

If you want to prevent unhappy evenings, consider easing your child's path throughout the daylight hours, especially at the height of separation anxiety.

Increasing predictability

One strategy for creating peace and quiet is to minimize changes. The following suggestions can assist you in minimizing your baby's daily stress:

Allow your kid to approach strangers, acquaintances, and family members on her own terms at home. This is most definitely not the moment to grab her up and say, "Give Nana a huge kiss!" (unless Nana is very adept at handling rejection). Rather than that, let your kid to quietly watch others and determine when she is ready to be more sociable.

Consistent nap times are best; prepare your little angel for naps with peaceful activities, lullabies, a story, and a cuddle.

Avoid switching sitters or day care providers if feasible throughout this stage of your child's life.

If you must leave a nervous toddler with a friend or sitter, make the goodbye pleasant. Say "Bye-bye, I'll see you soon," and slide away. Even if you're worried about leaving your sweetheart, keep a grin on your face until you're safely out of sight.

If at all possible, avoid taking a long vacation away from your kid at this stage of her life. A toddler's perception of time is imprecise, and even a lengthy weekend may feel ephemeral. While you may have earned some time off, the cost — in terms of restless nights — may be very high.

Making an informed preschool choice

To help your kid deal with separation anxiety, delay preschool until your child is closer to the age of two — when her language abilities and knowledge that you will return will assist her in coping. Children under the age of three

Frequently, when removed from a cherished caregiver, they exhibit intense emotions.

However, if preschool is a must, a child beyond the age of two may make this change with little grumbling. You may ease the transition by enrolling your kid in a preschool that allows for gradual transition. This means you get to remain with your little tot while she adjusts to her new instructors and surroundings. To learn more about sleep treatments that include day care, go forward to Section 11.

Dealing with interruptions to your routine

Even if your nighttime ritual is flawless, it is not always sufficient. Numerous little and large changes — a change in babysitters or the eruption of a new tooth — may create a stumbling block, and at times it seems as if you've taken a U-turn. When this happens, pause and reintroduce some of the techniques discussed in Section 5.

Refreshing Baby's memory: Recapitulating the fundamentals

If your child is regressing, be adamant about your nighttime routine in order to restore the fundamentals:

As you leave the room and your kid sobs or knocks on the crib bars, gently remark, "I love you." It's time to go to bed, and I'll see you in the morning." Then leave quietly and pleasantly, closing the door behind you.

Prepare yourself for your baby to cry for about 30 to 60 minutes.

Your kid is dissatisfied but unharmed; he desires but does not need you. (See Section 3 for a further discussion of these critical differences.) Make a concerted effort — a concerted effort! — to resist the temptation to return to his room, even if he says those new power words: "Mama!" and "Dada!"

If you are unable to refrain, enter quickly, pat him on the back, tell him once more how much you love him, and tell him you will see him in the morning.

Be gentle with yourself if you succumb and pay him a visit. However, keep in mind that every time your sweetheart wins a game, he wants to win it again. He's similar to a Vegas gambler, and you're the reward that keeps him pushing the lever.

At 12 a.m., striking a deal

If your kid falls asleep but then awakens throughout the night, you'll want to have a strategy in place (after all, who likes to start from scratch?).

Here are some methods for striking a balance between harsh love and complete surrender.

Maintain simplicity. Analyze your baby's screams to determine if he is really in distress or is just seeking attention. If you're certain there's nothing major, prepare to wait it out.

This delay method allows you (and your little Paul Revere) to determine if he is capable of falling asleep on his own. Allowing him to scream it out and console himself is the best course of action, although it is undoubtedly difficult. If you must enter his room for whatever reason, give him a brief touch and a comforting remark and then go. Avoid picking him up; else, you will indicate playtime. (Yikes!)

Maintain your composure. If a few minutes seems like an eternity and you can't resist the need to console your little howler, make a bargain with your softer side:

• If you hear your child crying at 12:02 a.m., remind yourself: "It's 12:02 a.m. now." I'll enter if he's still screaming at 12:15."

• At 12:15 p.m., reassess his cries. If they're still as loud, if not louder, and you're unable to take any more, approach him.

If you detect that he is winding down, however, establish a new goal time and see if he falls asleep before the new time.

Continue to increase the intervals. If he repeatedly wakes you up, make him wait a bit longer each time. If you wait ten minutes the first time, increase it to twenty the second time, and so on. Parents who use this method often discover that 45 minutes is the maximum amount of time they can wait before entering. However, after going in three or four times at ever-increasing intervals, you may want to just declare, "That's it, people," and stay out till dawn — even if your pride and joy screams for another hour.

This method soothes Mom and Dad, although it takes longer than staying out of your tot's room entirely. If you and your family are OK with the slower pace, it is a reasonable compromise.

Follow this procedure each time a problem arises in the middle of the night to ensure that you nip those pesky bugs in the bud. Over time, your child's wake-up calls will grow fewer and further between — and you'll gain confidence as you learn how establishing boundaries benefits both of you.

When Issues Recur: Keeping an Eye on Your Child's Sleep Patterns

The mix of separation anxiety, significant new abilities like as walking and talking, and more independence may make resolving sleep problems more difficult than ever at this time. To help make sense of the mayhem, consider replacing your hour-by-hour sleep record with the one in Table 6-1, which enables you to note clues such as life changes, the impact of new individuals in your tot's life, and significant milestones.

Sleep Log and Milestones			
Date	Duration of Sleep and/or Sleep	What's New? (Company Visiting	Mileston e Reached

	Problems Spotted	**New Sitter, and So On)**	
January 15 (4 m/o)	Night - 10 hrs.; woke up twice during the night; nap - 3 hrs.	Visit from Grandma	
March 23	Night - 9 hrs.; up at night 2-3x; nap - 2 hrs.	Back from vacation trip	
May 3	Night - 10 hrs.; up twice crying, clearly uncomfortable ; nap – 2hrs		Learning to stand
July 19 (10 m/o)	Night - 10 hrs.; had trouble falling asleep, very clingy; nap - 2 hrs.	Visit from Grandma	
August 12	Night - 10 hours; up once, fussy; nap - 2 hours		Took first step!
November 16	Night - 3 hours; nap - none	A bad cold	

Three Additional Success Strategies: Safety, Naps, and Substitutes

Once you've honed your sleep routine and dealt with separation anxiety, your evenings should once again be filled with pleasant dreams. However, you are not finished until you take three more measures to guarantee a secure and peaceful sleep time for everyone: Revise your safety guidelines; modify sleep times accordingly; and provide age-appropriate lovies and calming replacements for Mommy or Daddy.

Check for safety: Down the mattress, out the bumpers, and in the lovie!

Young toddlers have a strong case of wanderlust, so keep an eye out for ways for your little explorer to get into mischief throughout the night. When he reaches the standing stage, lower the crib mattress to the point where his head is barely over the crib rail. This height prevents him from climbing up and over the top rail, where he would have a terrible fall. Additionally, if you haven't previously removed the crib bumpers, do it now so they don't offer him a leg up... and out.

Nota bene: fantastic news on the safety front! After the first year, the risk of sudden infant death syndrome (SIDS) is very low, so you may breathe a sigh of relief and place your child's favorite blanket or stuffed animal in the cot with him. Simply ensure that the toys do not have sharp edges and are, of course, suitable for children under the age of two. (Also check that his toys do not have any loose pieces that he may put in his mouth or any holes that might allow stuffing to escape.)

Consolidating two naps

Most children tend to forego their morning sleep in favor of a lengthier afternoon nap somewhere during their second year of life. As you would imagine, this transformation does not occur overnight — and it may take some effort on your part!

The first sign is when your child refuses to nap in the morning or delays her nap until late morning and then sleeps poorly in the afternoon. These are indications that your baby's world is expanding; she is now capable of being awake for extended periods of time, taking in all the new sights and noises. While you may first miss the morning break (ideal for a short shower), you will quickly discover that a longer afternoon sleep provides both you and your angel with much-needed rest from a hectic day.

While some infants grasp this switch on their own, the majority need assistance:

Numerous infants seem to prefer to nap just before lunch - it's not unusual to discover a small toddler dozing off with her head resting on her macaroni and cheese! To prevent this, feed your toddler a little sooner by shifting the timetable up by 15 or 30 minutes (although some children may not eat as well as they should since breakfast is still fresh in their minds). If you do not feed her before to nap time, her stomach will wake her up and she will not be able to sleep as long as she should.

As your kid develops, feed her later and later until she eats at a time that is more convenient for her. Allow her a little pause before bedtime to allow nature to take its course (diaper-wise) and her stomach to relax.

Some parents discover that their kid is so eager for an afternoon nap that she sleeps for an extended period of time. Determine your child's sleep requirements, and if a prolonged nap does not conflict with a normal bedtime, go for it. However, you may discover that you must awaken your sleeping beauty in order to ensure a reasonable bedtime hour.

Updating your lovies to accommodate a separation-averse sweetheart

In Section 5, we discuss transitional objects, or lovies – things such as photographs or pieces of clothing that serve as a reminder of you to your cherub when you are not there. These may be effective aids throughout the separation anxiety period, and now that your angel is a bit older, you can be more creative.

For example, some parents purchase nontoxic ink stamps and create a little pattern — a butterfly, flower, or dinosaur, for example — on their child's arm, explaining, "That's exactly where I'm going to give you a big kiss when I pick you up today."

This is a fantastic concept since, unlike lovies, an ink stamp cannot be misplaced (place the stamp in an inaccessible location – not on a hand!). Allow your kid to choose several stamps to add to the excitement — and maybe allow her to stamp you as well.

Section 7

The Awakening: Sleep Between 18 Months and 2 Years

Throughout This Section...

- ➢ Observing your youngster as she explores her new environment
- ➢ Recognize a child's nocturnal fantasies
- ➢ Eliminating the midnight bottle and leaving the crib

If toddlers had an official slogan as they neared their second birthday, it would be: "Watch out, world, here I am — but where am I!" After spending the first year and a half in a cocoon of comfort, with Mommy or Daddy meeting every need, they've reached a new level of awareness. As with butterflies, they are emerging to take on new perspectives on their environment.

Not surprisingly, this major transition, along with the numerous
other physical and mental changes associated with this age
(such as giving up the nighttime bottle and transitioning from
crib to big bed, which we discuss near the end of this Section),
can have an unexpected effect on your tot's sleep cycle.
Additionally, this Section discusses several typical sleep
disorders that occur during this time period: nightmares, night
terrors, sleep-talking, and sleepwalking. Additionally, two
frightening but usually harmless nighttime habits are described:
rocking and headbanging. (No, this is not a toddler rave; this is a
natural developmental period!) Additionally, we take a brief
look at teeth grinding, an annoyance that is often transitory.

Changes in the 1¹/₂-Year-Old

The age of twelve is a period of rapid transformation. While
your 12-month-old and 20-month-old may seem to be same on
the surface, the inside is very different.

Only adolescence results in such significant changes, and
parents often know what to anticipate (and fear!) when their
child reaches puberty. However, the dramatic changes that
occur in an 18-month-old infant often catch families by surprise.
Thus, anticipating what to anticipate may help you stay one step
ahead – particularly when sleep is at risk.

Increasing awareness

Consciousness — or, as some like to call it, the awareness of consciousness — is the most amazing feature of human existence, and it starts at this age. Previously, your baby was aware of a hungry stomach or a damp diaper, but now she is aware of her awareness. She is cultivating a mental life, which enables her to contemplate huge issues like "What am I really yearning for?" This is a significant milestone – the largest since birth.

The strength of this new awareness is also its greatest limitation. For the remainder of your child's life, every circumstance will provide a chance to consider, "How might this be improved?" When she learns that nighttime does not have to be the way it has always been, for example, her well-established sleep patterns become targets.

Appropriately arousing desire and imagination

Until recently, your kid seemed to be very content with life. His eyes, on the other hand, are now open to the vast and fascinating world around him, and this knowledge fuels an expanding imagination and a strong new emotion: desire.

However, due to his poor communication abilities, he is unable to make sense of or communicate these emotions.

Consider the following three emotions and how they create new obstacles:

The infantile imagination: The capacity to create a mental picture of something that is not physically there is referred to as imagination. Your child is no longer happy to play with the toy in his hand, read a storybook on the sofa, or eat cookies from the kitchen cabinet.

Desire's strength: This little guy is aware that there is an abundance of beautiful and fantastic things available, and he wants it all – immediately, immediately, immediately. This rush of want may be overpowering, particularly when coupled with the new and nagging sense that the here-and-now isn't good enough. He is aware that he wants something unique, but he is unsure of what he desires or how to get it.

Communication abilities are limited: With time, as your toddler's vocabulary expands, he will be able to more readily express his ideas and desires. However, not at the age of 18 months! At the moment, he is a bundle of raging passions that he cannot articulate – to himself or to you.

That is why you are seeing your first glimpses of the approaching dreadful twos.

These overpowering emotions result in some rather severe sleep disruptions, which we will discuss in more detail in the next section. They also explain why you're experiencing certain new sleep problems at this age.

What to Expect During Sleepy Time from the Active Mind?

Once upon a time (indeed, only a few weeks ago), your baby slept peacefully. The road to dreamland was rather treacherous, but once there, your darling slept well. Now she is evolving, and her increased consciousness and creativity have the potential to transform the once-peaceful Land of Nod into dangerous territory.

Several behaviors that you may have seen in previous months may become more regular or severe at this period. They include the following:

- ➢ Before sleep, rocking and head-banging
- ➢ During sleep, teeth grinding
- ➢ Nightmares and terrors of the night
- ➢ Sleepwalking and sleep-talking are both common occurrences.

While some of these behaviors may seem frightening, nocturnal thrills and shivers are nearly usually typical throughout the toddler years. As long as your toddler is happy and well-adjusted throughout the day, there is no need for you to be concerned or guilty – the overwhelming majority of these issues have nothing to do with home, school, or you.

If you want a firm grasp of the hows and whys of the sleep events discussed in the next sections, we suggest starting with Section 2. If, on the other hand, you'd prefer cut to the point and receive some short tips on how to deal with each habit, continue reading.

There is a great deal of shaking going on!

Head-banging and

rocking

It may be frightening to see your little angel whacking his head against the crib bars or headboard just after tuck-in time. However, do not worry if this occurs; head-banging and its close cousin, cribrocking, are both frequent and acceptable behaviors in this age range. Indeed, about one in every six toddlers rocks or head-bangs. Nota bene: The acts may begin before or after the age of 18 months, but they often cease by the age of two.

The reason for rocking and head-banging is straightforward: Both acts are really relaxing. There is a world of difference between a toddler's busy, action-packed daily hours and the peaceful condition of just lying there. This is a method for some little nippers to drain their batteries before snuggling down for the night.

Both of these behaviors may be very worrisome to parents, who usually inquire four times. The following list includes the following questions, along with our responses and explanations:

Is it possible for my kid to injure himself when he head-bangs? No. Rocking and even head-banging come dangerously close to inflicting injury.

While safeguarding those little noggins is critical, headbanging in bed does not harm them.

Is he acting in this manner because he is enraged about something? If your kid seems to be happy and well-adjusted throughout the day, rocking and head banging are not indicative of emotional distress.

However, if your child seems uncomfortable or disturbed during waking hours, contact his doctor immediately. The problem at hand is daytime concerns, not rocking and head-banging in bed.

Is this an early warning sign that he may have a health problem? While rocking and head-banging may trigger a parent's suspicions that their kid is developing abnormally, the determining element is the quality of interaction during the day, not the rocking and head-banging before sleep.

Should parents intervene to prevent their child from headbanging in bed? No, for two very excellent reasons. One: There is little you can do to change this habit. Two: There is no damage being done, so why should it be stopped?

If your child is social, readily establishes eye contact, reacts when spoken to, and is generally on pace with key developmental milestones, don't fret about these common-as-dirt nighttime habits.

Grinding the chompers is the tooth fairy's pet dislike?

The sound of a child grinding her teeth in her sleep (also known as bruxism) is similar to the sound of fingernails on a chalkboard — only worse, since it increases the worry that she may wear her pearly whites down to a nubbin.

Fortunately, these concerns are without merit. Tooth grinding, it turns out, is a perfectly common and innocuous habit at this age.

Doctors have no idea why some children grind their teeth and others do not. Some specialists believe it has to do with repositioning the teeth, while others believe it is a method of expressing emotions.

Around one in every five children is a teeth grinder, although the habit often fades away as children go beyond their early childhood years. Adults and older children should be concerned – yet toddlers seem unconcerned.

If you're concerned about your child's teeth being damaged, have her dentist examine to see if the enamel is worn away or if any teeth have chips or cracks. Additionally, inquire as to if your child's jaw aches. Neither the dentist nor your kid will most likely report any issues.

Our recommendation? Assure yourself that, although this activity may be unpleasant to your ears, it is not harmful to your toddler's teeth. Cross this concern off your list... and turn on your MP3 player to avoid hearing that horrible noise!

Diverse issues, divergent solutions: Nightmares and terrors of the night

At 3 a.m., you jump out of bed and sprint to your toddler's bedside. He's sitting up in bed, screaming uncontrollably, and you're wondering, "How can I assist?"

This question has two possible solutions, and in order to choose the correct one, you must first determine which situation you are watching. Is this a dream or a night terror? They may seem and sound identical, but they are as unlike as night and day — and their respective methods for coping with them.

We will explain why in the next sections.

Nightmares: The pernicious aspect of dreaming

We discuss rapid-eye-movement (REM) sleep in Section 2, the period during which individuals experience vivid dreams. A nightmare is just a dream, but one that is filled with negative emotions such as dread and sorrow. As with every other dream, it contains two intriguing characteristics:

It feels very genuine.

Individuals often recall it upon awakening.

Indeed, dreams (both pleasant and unpleasant) seem to be entirely about recollection.

Dreams are constructed from the components of our waking experiences; in turn, they construct their own memories that may carry over into the day. However, negative memories are more potent because fear and sorrow are so very strong. While life is full of pleasures, it also contains pain and loss. Unfortunately, as consciousness develops at the age of 18 months, a tot's knowledge of what may go wrong develops as well. This offers some frightening new plotlines to your child's nightmares.

Children's dreams may be much more vivid and frightening than those of adults. Toddlers have an awareness of the hazards in the world at this age – people get injured, flowers perish, and Mommy and Daddy may become ill. As a consequence, a child's negative memories are often very vivid. Even the happiest little children go to bed carrying hefty baggage (memories) of actual and imagined concerns, which may manifest in their dreams.

What should you do if your kid awakens crying after a terrible dream? Bear the following ideas in mind:

1. Ascertain that he is really experiencing a nightmare and not a night terror (see the next section).

If it is a nightmare, he will remain awake but will attempt to determine whether reality is real — the land of dreams or his secure bedroom.

2. Assist him in returning to reality by soothing him, explaining that dreams are not real, and being with him until he realizes that everything is OK.

Your touch, your voice, the sight of your face, and even your familiar scent all contribute to his recovery from his frightening experience.

Night terrors: Deep sleep's perilous journey

While night terrors are one of the most frightening occurrences a parent can see, they are also very typical — which may comfort a mom or dad witnessing the frightening incident. They are the most prevalent.

Often occurs in children between the ages of $1^1/_2$ and 3, affecting up to 5% of toddlers in this age range.

To comprehend night terrors, it's necessary to grasp how they vary from nightmares in terms of their underlying origins and symptoms:

They occur at the following times: Night terrors occur during sleep arousals, short periods of consciousness during deep sleep, which correspond to the Stage 4 discussed in Section 2. On the other hand, nightmares occur on the verge of awakening during REM sleep.

How they influence your toddler's sleeping behavior: Night terrors cause a sleeper's body to behave as if he is awake; in contrast, a person's body does not move during nightmares.

A child suffering from a night nightmare may play out the scenario unfolding in his sound-asleep mind. For instance, he may leap and scream at the top of his lungs in his crib.

They have an effect on one's capacity to wake up: While a kid experiencing a night terror is sound asleep and often difficult to arouse (due to being in Stage 4 sleep), a parent can rouse a child from a nightmare — and a terrible dream may even startle him up.

They have an effect on your toddler's waking life in the following ways: Individuals experiencing night terrors often have no awareness or recollection of the experience, while nightmares are commonly recalled.

To sleep, to dream... but why?

When we dream, our brains conjure up scenarios that feel real.

However, what is the purpose of this? What possible benefit could there be in winning the lottery or sinking a three-pointer in the NBA finals if they occur only in our imaginations?

Freud, the most eminent dream analyst, believed that dreams enable our brains to break free from the rules and constraints of our awake hours, allowing us to experience life without boundaries. As a result, he speculated, we get the opportunity to experiment with alternative approaches to problems without incurring the consequences of real-world decisions.

A very different theory emerges from contemporary neuroscience, which proposes that dreams aid in the repair of the wear and tear on our brains caused by daily life.

According to this line of thought, dreams construct or repair the circuits that enable us to recall the day's most critical life lessons. If this theory is correct, dreams provide an opportunity for our brains to conduct dress rehearsals, allowing our memories to become firmly established. And, in the case of toddlers, who are constantly forming thousands of new brain circuits, establishing these memories is essential!

If you mistake a night terror for a nightmare, you anticipate your screaming toddler leaping into your arms upon your arrival at his bedside. In reality, he is unaware of your presence, even if his eyes are wide open and you are directly in front of him! This is a highly distressing situation for a loving parent who is attempting to rescue a toddler from a terrifying event.

Your child is just as asleep during a night terror as he is when he is dozing blissfully. As a result, your reassuring words and embraces have no effect whatsoever.

What are your options for dealing with your shrieking, crib-rattling, unable-to-wake-up toddler? Our advice is to take no action at all for the following reasons:

You cannot rouse your sweetheart while he or she is having a night terror.

The episode concludes shortly thereafter, and your child snuggles back down to sleep peacefully once more.

In the morning, when you're bleary-eyed, he'll have no idea what happened. When night terrors pass, they typically leave no trace.

When you recognize a night terror for what it is, you will be able to relax regardless of how bloodthirsty your little bedbug is screaming.

You'll recognize that this is a harmless phenomenon associated with very deep sleep that does not persist upon awakening.

The only exception to the do-nothing strategy is for children who experience night terrors nearly every night at the same time.

If this is the case in your household, you can attempt to disrupt the sleep cycle by waking your child half an hour or an hour before night terror hour arrives.

Aspects of a theme: Sleepwalking and sleep-talking are both common occurrences

It serves as the basis for a number of beloved stories: Mom or Dad hears a strange noise in the night and ventures out to discover Junior raiding the refrigerator or pooping on the potty while completely unconscious. In other versions, parents discover their small children mumbling or even speaking in sentences while sleeping.

These behaviors, dubbed sleepwalking and sleep-talking, occur during sleep arousals, just as night terrors do. Toddlers' brains are functioning normally during these arousals.

While their bodies are asleep, they can still move — and occasionally venture off on their own adventures in the middle of the night.

Sleep-talking is extremely common — approximately one-third of toddlers engage in it — and it becomes even more prevalent as children enter their preteen years. Sleepwalking, on the other hand, is more common, affecting approximately one-tenth of children by age ten. Neither behavior is cause for alarm as long as a sleepwalker can be safely corralled.

Knowing the duration of these disturbances

Numerous sleepwalking episodes and nearly all sleep-talking episodes are brief. For instance, while snoozing, your little cuddle-bunny may murmur a few gibberish syllables or stand up next to the bed for a few seconds before collapsing again.

Toddlers' sleep-talking or sleepwalking episodes can last several minutes in some cases. Sleepwalking toddlers may perform several extremely complex steps before doing something completely out of character. For instance, a child may rise confidently from bed, walk confidently to the closet, pull down her pants, pee on the floor, and march back to bed efficiently.

Appropriate response

If your little sweet cake is a sleep-talker, there is no point in attempting to translate her messages. Rather than being a child's attempt to communicate a deeply felt emotion, sleep-talking is typically just meaningless strings of nonsense. Sleep-talking is not a window into the soul, unless your child's soul is attempting to communicate, "Wubba tubba gicky boo!"

On the other hand, the dangers of sleepwalking are not amusing, nor is the distress it can cause parents. When a small sleepwalker begins to walk, all manner of mischief can ensue. For example, many parents recount horror stories about their toddlers opening the front door and taking a stroll around the neighborhood in their pajamas. A brief episode of sleepwalking, on the other hand, is nothing to be concerned about — just keep the following tips in mind:

Avoid attempting to awaken your child while she is sleepwalking. As with night terrors, she is in a deep state of sleep and nearly impossible to awaken. If she does not resist, gently guide her back to bed — but do not attempt to coerce her.

When your child is awake, avoid discussing sleepwalking with her. She has no control over it and will typically have no memory of it when she awakens, so you will only cause her anxiety and make it more difficult for her to fall asleep.

If your toddler has developed a sleepwalking habit, continue reading for our advice.

Maintaining the safety of a sleepwalker

If you witness repeated instances of sleepwalking, you must take extra precautions to keep your little sugar plum safe. Prior to modifying your home in general, confine your child to her bedroom and ensure the safety of her immediate surroundings:

Install a toddler gate at the bedroom door to contain your free-roaming toddler. The gate creates a barrier between your child and the rest of the house and family without isolating him or her.

Ascertain that all bedroom floor coverings are slip-resistant (and machine-washable in the event of a pee incident!).

Cushion sharp corners.

Ascertain that all outlets are childproof, preferably with a back plate that prevents anything other than a plug from being inserted.

Each night, view the room through the eyes of a child, noting anything your child might come into contact with while moving in an unpredictable manner. Remove toys from the floor to prevent her from tripping over them, and keep breakables out of her reach.

After ensuring the safety of the bedroom, secure the rest of your home's entrances:

Secure the doors leading to the stairs and install baby gates in areas where the stairs lack doors.

Keep exterior door locks out of reach of your toddler.

Consider installing a motion-activated alarm that activates when an exterior door is opened.

Smoothing At This Age, There Are Two Significant Transitions

Toddlers begin their march toward preschool age between the ages of $1^1/_2$ and 2. As your toddler matures and gains independence, he gradually abandons his infant ways.

Two significant steps in that direction are as follows: transitioning from bottles or even regular nursing to a cup.

Making the transition from a crib or your bed to a big kid bed.

If your child is accustomed to a nighttime bottle, the transition to a cup may cause a hiccup in your sleepy-time routine. The transition to a larger bed can upend the beddy-bye routine and raise critical safety concerns.

Bye-bye, bedtime bottle

If your infant is bottle-fed (breastfeeding parents may skip this section), the time will come when you will decide to transition to a cup. You're likely to abandon the daytime bottles first, followed by the nighttime bottles.

At this stage, the bedtime bottle is a favorite of your child, and it has been an integral part of the bedtime ritual up to this point. Therefore, when the time comes to say good-bye, be prepared for some sleepy-time fallout.

Before you remove the nighttime bottle, you must pique your child's interest in the bottle's contents. Simply put, you want to detract from the bottle's contents. This preparatory phase ensures that your toddler will not go hungry when the bottle is finished. Take the following steps:

1. Ascertain that your infant is capable of drinking from a cup. You don't want to ask your sweetie to perform an action she is incapable of performing.

(For more information, see the preceding section, "Knowing When to Give It Up.")

2. Begin gradually diluting the bottle's contents with water. For example, switch to 18-ounce water for two to three days, then to 14-ounce water for another two to three days, and finally to a 50-50 mixture of water and formula or breast milk for two to three days.

3. Repeat the dilution strategy until the bottle is completely filled with water. Nota bene: We do not recommend introducing juice into your diet because it has been shown to cause excessive weight gain.

Now, simply wait for the appropriate time to discontinue providing the bedtime bottle entirely — preferably when no other significant life changes occur and your child's sleep patterns are stable. (Since giving up the bedtime bottle creates a significant hole in your toddler's nighty-night routine, you'll want to ensure that the rest of the ritual remains intact.) If you do not already have a bedtime routine, Section 5 contains suggestions for developing one.

When the nighttime bottle is removed, your child will miss it, will feel sad or angry for a short period of time, and will fuss the first few nights. You can be understanding, kind, and loving in response — but whatever you do,

Do not return the bottle! In lieu of that, offer a cup of water. After all, as long as you maintain your composure, this brief cloudburst will pass in a day or two.

The transition from crib

to big bed

Just as no one drinks from a baby bottle indefinitely, no one stays in a crib indefinitely. However, the case of cribs versus beds raises a significant safety concern: jumping from a crib can result in broken bones.

> ➢ Therefore, ensure that you make the necessary changes before that risk becomes a reality.
> ➢ This section will assist you in making this transition safely and successfully.
> ➢ Identifying the optimal time to make the switch

The first priority is to keep your toddler safe. Therefore, if your child is bouncing around the crib, clinging to the bars like a monkey, or attempting somersaults over the top rail, consider transitioning him from the crib to a grownup bed. And if your toddler is actually attempting to climb out of the crib, make the transition quickly — before he takes a potentially fatal tumble.

On the other hand, if your toddler is content to remain in the crib (and you are certain he cannot jump out), the timing is somewhat more flexible. In any case, we recommend initiating the transition at the age of 18 months. If you choose to wait much longer than this age, transition your child from the crib to the bed before beginning toilet training. The big bed serves as a signal to your child that he is maturing and prepares him for other significant milestones, such as using the potty.

The optimal time for the crib-to-bed transition is determined not only by your toddler's climbing ability, but also by what is going on in his world. Two issues that may influence your decision are as follows:

Are you expecting a child who will require a crib? If the stork is due to visit soon, transition your toddler to a big bed at least six to eight weeks prior to the arrival of your new baby. Consider completely dismantling the crib with the assistance of your child and storing it until you're ready for your new arrival. This way, your child is less likely to believe he is being kicked out solely to make way for his new sibling to take over his territory.

Are there any other significant changes occurring in your child's life? Make this transition during a relatively calm period in your toddler's life.

Leaving his secure, small crib may be too much for him to bear if he is also coping with significant life changes, such as an illness or a move to a new home. Additionally, defer the crib-to-bed transition if your child is currently undergoing toilet training, a good motto to live by is: One significant change at a time.

The bed is introduced

When the new bed becomes available, prepare your toddler for the transition. Discuss how exciting it is that he is ready for this mature step and take him to the store to assist you in selecting new sheets and pillows. You could even create a picture book to commemorate this momentous occasion (see Section 14 for ideas). Additionally, if you begin by placing the crib mattress on the floor (see the subsequent section "Making the move"), the transition will be so subtle that your sweetie will likely not object at all.

Preparing the room

When the crib is no longer necessary, your toddler has complete control of his room at night. A thorough safety inspection is required at this point! When your child begins crawling or walking, the following childproofing steps should already be in place, but now is a good time to review them:

1. Ensure that all outlet covers are secure — not the small plastic ones that your child can pull out and swallow.

2. Remove any furniture that is susceptible to being knocked over by a child (or secure it to the wall).

3. Secure dresser drawers with locks to prevent your small wanderer from using them as stepping stones.

4. Secure the closet door with a latch.

5. Hide drapery pulls, pictures, and mobiles.

6. Teach your child to put away his toys prior to bedtime to avoid tripping over them if he awakens during the night.

Additionally, when the crib no longer restricts nighttime journeys, take the following steps:

A door gate should be installed.

This effectively converts the room into a crib and prevents your child from wandering around the house at night. Ascertain that the gate is sturdy enough to prevent your toddler from pushing it open.

Include a nightlight to ensure your munchkin's safety in the dark.

Making the transition

When the time comes to transition your baby to the big bed, follow these steps to ensure a smooth transition:

1. Begin with the crib-on-the-floor method.

Beginning your baby's life on his crib mattress has two significant advantages. To begin, he is safe because crib mattresses are only a few inches high; falling is unlikely to result in injury or even arousal. Second, this is the mattress your child is familiar with and loves, and its familiar feel and smell help to mitigate the drama associated with this significant change.

To begin, place the crib mattress on the floor for daytime naps and then replace it in the crib at night. When your child becomes accustomed to sleeping outside the crib bars, you can also leave the mattress on the floor at night. Remove the crib at this point. (Allow your angel to observe and even assist a little, so he does not believe it vanished into thin air!)

2. Once your sweetie has a firm grasp on his new boundaries, switch the crib mattress for the bed mattress you intend to use in the long run.

Simply place the new mattress flat on the floor once more. It's simple to determine when to do this; simply wait until your child stays on the crib mattress for an uninterrupted one to two weeks without rolling off onto the floor.

3. Add the box frame once your child appears to be at ease on the new mattress and has gone one to two weeks without spilling anything on the floor.

4. After your child has been fall-free for another one to two weeks, complete the ensemble by adding the bed frame.

Fortunately, the risk of SIDS has been eliminated completely by the time your child reaches his first birthday, which means he can sleep on his back, stomach, or even his head! Additionally, he may possess a variety of sheets, blankets, pillows, and stuffed animals. Toddler beds can also be placed anywhere in the room, so feel free to use a wall to prevent falls.

Managing free-roaming children

At the toddler stage, an odd thing occurs: Parents who did not co-sleep with their infant begin to hear the sound of freedom — the pitter-patter of tiny feet making their way to the master bedroom.

If your toddler begins invading your territory as he moves from crib to bed, see Section 8 for suggestions on how to keep him in his own room. Of course, another option is to scoot over and invite him to join you. Whichever course of action you take, be consistent! If you choose to begin co-sleeping at this stage, ensure that it is your choice, not your toddler's.

Section 8

The Great Tug of War: Sleep Between the Ages of 2 and 3 Years

Throughout This Section_

- ➢ Observing your child's changing emotions
- ➢ Preparing for bedtime and dealing with your unwilling sleeper
- ➢ Saying Farewell to Naps
- ➢ Confronting your child's fears about the nighttime potty

One stage of childhood more than any other requires saintly patience and steely nerves — the phase parents affectionately refer to as the Terrible Twos. At this point, your infant is no longer a baby, and his new abilities are becoming increasingly complex on a daily basis. These changes are both exciting and distressing to him. And a toddler expresses on the outside what he feels on the inside.

Despite the strain that these twelve months can impose, we prefer the term tumultuous rather than terrible. As your child's world expands in exciting ways, he experiences an emotional roller coaster — and you get to ride along for the ride. As a result, both of you will experience plenty of ups and downs, but it will be an incredible period of growth, discovery, and maturation.

You will have several sleepless nights during this ride as your toddler attempts to cope with real and imagined fears, gives up naps, and masters the art of peeing and pooping in the night hours. However, by following the advice in this Section, you can help him adjust to these changes while also alleviating his fears and anxieties.

With any luck, you'll discover that sleep is not a fantasy!

A Sneak Peek at Your

Child's Issues at This Age

Numerous changes occur within your infant as she grows from infancy to childhood, and her ever-growing brain provides her with a more sophisticated perspective on life. For instance, she has a rudimentary grasp of time and is aware that you have not completely vanished even when you are not physically present. In some ways, she resembles a tween — no longer a baby but not quite a small child.

She struggles with abandoning her baby ways, unsure that being big is all it's cracked up to be. (Diapers do appear to be a lot more convenient than remembering to use the restroom!)

Children at this age truly understand their separation from their parents, but this awareness does not automatically transform them into Gandhi or Mother Theresa. On the other hand, the theme song for this era could be "I've Gotta Be Me!" with the subtitle "It's All About Me." Although egocentric is not a term that one would use to describe an adult, it is an apt (and perfectly normal) description of a toddler.

Recognize your toddler's internal struggle

Do any of the following scenarios ring a bell?

On days when you're pressed for time, your toddler insists on putting on his own shoes. On other days, when you have all the time in the world, your sweetheart collapses to the floor and cries, "You do it!"

You're at a friend's birthday party, and your toddler is clingy as lint to you. He's as slippery as an eel just a few hours later at the mall.

No wonder this era has such a bad reputation! To comprehend this stage of development and its impact on your toddler's sleep habits, you must first understand what your toddler is thinking and feeling as he transitions from one mood to the next.

Consider your child in a tug-of-war with himself. The baby inside him is pulling on one end of the rope, while the big boy is tugging on the other. The big-boy side will eventually win, but the momentum in this tug of war is shifting from moment to moment.

This contradictory behavior can be perplexing and perplexing for parents because adults analyze situations rationally — something your toddler cannot do at the moment. For instance, your child may say "No" to something he normally enjoys or anticipates. Why?

It's his way of expressing himself and his desire for independence — while still desiring your leadership.

Observing how a two-year-emotions old's affect his or her sleep

Every aspect of your toddler's life is affected by the conflict between baby and big person, and sleep is no exception. That is why a toddler who slept peacefully for months may now appear each night like a Jack-in-the-Box.

However, why would a two-year-old fight a nap when she is so exhausted, she can barely stand? (How delightful it would be if someone told you to go lie down!)

Here are a few observations:

The world is more magical than logical to your toddler. This mixture of real and unreal feelings can easily obstruct the process of letting go and falling asleep.

Your infant is also concerned. Your toddler may comprehend just enough of a situation or change in her life to keep her awake. To a toddler, the world revolves around them, and thus anything that happens in that world is naturally their fault. If Mommy and Daddy quarrel or Grandma becomes ill, for example, they must be the cause. This way of thinking can easily clog the sleep mechanism.

Children of this age continue to view you as omnipotent and capable of fixing anything. We know of one child who was enraged at her mother for being unable to stop the rain! As your child's world becomes more logical, she may feel a little uncertain: "How can everything be okay if Mom and Dad can't make everything better all the time?" This new concern has the potential to infiltrate small minds and disrupt sleep.

Your toddler has difficulty seeing the world through your eyes. When she calls in the middle of the night, she fully anticipates your arrival to repair everything. Even though she is as sharp as a whip, she is unaware of the disruption her actions cause to your sleep; she simply wants you when she wants you.

At this age, your child is brimming with desires and oblivious to boundaries. If one cookie is delectable, six cookies dipped in ice cream are even more so! All logic in the world will not dispel this belief, and the same is true of wake-up calls: She can never have enough of them.

In short, your toddler is simply doing her job — maturing! And, like teenagers, 2-year-olds go through a stage in which contradictions, uncontrollable desires, and negativity are completely normal. (Of course, we did not say enjoyable; we said ordinary.)

In reality, the reason your child woke up and called for you has nothing to do with her requests. Yes, people get thirsty in the middle of the night and teddy bears go missing — but it's a safe bet that your toddler wants nothing more than you and is willing to push all of your buttons to get it!

If you fall for this trap, sleepy time will creep later and later each night, and those middle-of-the-night demands will become increasingly insistent. Even small children have an uncanny ability to wield power, and once she sees the effect her words have on you, she'll keep coming up with new ways to get you out of bed. While comprehending your child's emotional roller coaster may provide insight into sleep issues, these issues should not give your angel carte blanche over the routine. You can still exert control over your sleeping situation.

Promoting Sleep with Compassion While Standing Your Ground

Fortunately, you already have some tools in your bedtime toolbox. By implementing them firmly, lovingly, and consistently, you can rein in nighttime demands and reclaim control of your sleepy-time routine.

While you cannot force your child to sleep, you can prepare him for bed, provide him with a comfortable and safe sleeping environment, and expect him to stay in his room. Of course, achieving that final objective is easier said than done! However, fear not — this section will teach you how to effectively respond to your little escape artist.

Preparing for bedtime with the assistance of your toddler

Bedtime is an ideal time for parents to assist their children with their internal tug-of-war (see the previous section). A two-year-old is hungry to conquer the universe, and parents can assist by tugging on the rope's big-kid end while leaving the baby end alone. Your nighttime rituals so that your child is fully aware of what to expect and her role.

Instilling a sense of control in your child

Children of this age adore routines, and if you miss a step, your tot will undoubtedly point it out! Each night, clearly defined steps assist in winding down your infant and preparing her for sleep — both physically and emotionally. Additionally, by delegating some bedtime routines to your child, you give her a sense of control.

For example, parents can delegate some decisions to their child, such as what to wear, which book to read, or which toothpaste to use. These straightforward tasks send a strong message: It's time for bed, and you're big enough to prepare yourself! Additionally, purchase a digital clock for your toddler so that you can refrain from saying, "It's time for bed," and instead allow your toddler to communicate with you when sleepy time arrives. This technique frequently elicits easier compliance from toddlers during tuck-in time and enables them to take another step toward independent problem-solving — a critical life skill.

Appropriately addressing your child's learning style

Consider your approach as you assist your toddler in establishing a healthy sleep schedule. Adults, like children, have a variety of learning styles. Certain toddlers respond best to verbal cues (speech) and will readily follow along with their parents as they go through the bedtime routine. Others are triggered by visual or tactile cues (touch).

A schedule strip is one of the most effective methods for visual or tactile learners. How to create one is as follows:

Maintain a consistent bedtime routine that includes bathing, tooth brushing, putting on jammies, reading a bedtime story, and sleeping.

Divide the routine into four to six sections. Then, for each activity, draw a picture, cut out a magazine photo, or use a photograph of your child. (See Figure 8-1 for an illustration.)

In the evening, hand the strip to your child and ask her to predict the next activity. This alters the dynamic because she is now telling you what she is going to do next, rather than you telling her.

Keeping the upper hand when your child refuses to lie down

A significant challenge in assisting older toddlers in falling asleep is managing their desire to leave their room. (If this has not yet occurred, see Section 7 for instructions on how to transition from crib to bed.) If your toddler refuses to stay put after being tucked in, you have several options:

Install a sturdy gate, effectively converting his entire room into a large crib. Learn to ignore your child's pleas to leave, and don't be surprised if he spends the first few days sleeping on the floor rather than in his bed.

If a gate does not contain your small wanderer (for example, he is nimble enough to climb over it or undo the latch), return him to his room each time he leaves and inform him that you will close the door if he does not stay.

Nota bene: This works only if he sleeps with the door open.

If he continues to open the door, close it, signal to him that you are on the other side, and demonstrate that you mean business. Allow it to remain open only when he is able to remain in the room.

This strategy frequently succeeds, but it may backfire if he believes he is winning because you are still nearby. (If this occurs, abandon this strategy.)

Arrange books and quiet toys throughout the room. "I understand you don't feel like sleeping, but it's bedtime, and you can play by yourself until you do feel sleepy," explain to your toddler. Once again, this gives him some control over when he sleeps, which may help him be more cooperative.

Some families take a completely different approach, allowing their toddlers access to their room and allowing them to sleep in the adult bed or on the floor in a sleeping bag or blanket. This arrangement works well if you don't mind your bedroom resembling a youth hostel, but it can cause friction between partners who value their privacy. Additionally, if you or your partner are annoyed or resentful about sharing your space, your toddler is likely to pick up on those negative vibes.

If you choose this arrangement, you should anticipate that your child will remain your roommate until you take steps to rectify the situation. Children rarely return to their own room in these circumstances without a gentle nudge from Mom and Pop.

If your child is rapidly approaching the age of three and is still in his crib, you must assist him in transitioning to a big kid bed. Naturally, once your child is capable of jumping from a crib (even if he appears uninterested), safety dictates that he be moved to a bed. Section 7 contains additional information about this significant relocation.

Managing the Transitions

of a Two-Year-Old

There are so many changes! There is so little time! When your baby was a newborn, the changes were both physical and visibly noticeable. They may be less visible as your baby grows into a toddler, but they are just as real. Change is difficult for adults as well, so it's unsurprising that giving up the crib or diapers can send your pumpkin into a tailspin.

Choosing the order of transitions: Crib-to-bed transition or diapers-to-underpants transition?

If your toddler is still in the crib at the time of potty training, you must decide which change to make first. The simple answer is to transition your toddler from the crib to a bed first, as the crib represents infanthood and potty training represents a transition into a more adult phase.

Typically, baby books suggest the same progression. (In fact, that is why Section 7 discusses the crib transition.) However, the issue is that toddlers do not read baby books. As a result, you may end up with a toddler who is making great strides with toilet training but is unwilling to give up those crib bars.

If your child is more concerned with using the potty than with having a big girl bed, wait until her potty skills are firmly established before attempting to change her sleeping arrangements. Diapering and giving up the crib are two significant changes; implementing both at the same time can be overwhelming. Again, safety comes first, so if she is capable of climbing out of the crib, remove her first. (For details, see Section 7.)

When your napster sings his own tune in resolving nap issues

If your small child falls asleep in the afternoon (for example, in the car seat on the way home from the store), his afternoon nap can completely disrupt his nighttime sleep; even a 15-minute nap can keep him going at whirling-dervish speeds well past his usual bedtime. On the other hand, if you keep him awake until late afternoon, he may fall asleep around dinner time and then be ready to party until the early hours of the morning.

This section will walk you through the nap transition to assist you in avoiding these less-than-desirable situations.

Recognize when to discontinue the napping routine

While some toddlers nap until kindergarten, children frequently stop napping between the ages of two and three. This adjustment is frequently gradual but not always straightforward.

Indeed, at some point, you're likely to have an exhausted toddler who struggles mightily to sleep and ends the day as cranky as a wet mule.

There is no one-size-fits-all answer to the question of when your child should stop napping. A child who is resistant to napping but appears to disintegrate by late afternoon could probably benefit from some rest (see the next section for some ideas on how to structure one). However, you may want to eliminate daytime naps if your child's lengthy afternoon nap has a detrimental effect on his nighttime sleep, keeping him awake until 9, 10, or later. In this case, you may be willing to tolerate a cranky, demanding toddler for a few afternoon hours in exchange for a reasonable bedtime hour.

Assisting your infant during the transition

Toddlers are certain to experience some rough days when they give up naps, and you may feel powerless to prevent them. However, the following tips may prove useful:

Avoid late afternoon car rides and other calming activities. Road trips (even small ones!) and watching television on a soft couch predispose a child to a late-afternoon nap, so avoid these activities if you're attempting to keep your toddler awake.

In the late afternoon, plan an interesting activity. Consider baking cookies, creating an artwork, or whipping up some homemade play dough.

Feed your child earlier in the evening than usual, even if this means missing family dinners. While family mealtimes are critical, it is prudent to be flexible during this brief transitional period.

Arrange for your child's bedtime to be earlier. A toddler who has decided to forego his nap may go to bed as early as 7 p.m. and sleep until morning.

If you have a nanny or other caregiver in your home, delegate the preliminary tasks — bathing, tooth brushing, and so on — to your caregiver while you focus on other family responsibilities.

After that, you can take over for story time and cuddles. This plan enables you to advance your bedtime routine while still spending ample quality time with your sweetie. (See Section 10 for additional suggestions on how to approach this situation.)

Avoid being too concerned if these tricks do not work (and we can almost guarantee that they will not work every time). Even if you do everything possible to keep your toddler awake until bedtime, he is likely to fall asleep early and wake up too early at least a few times a week. Inconsistent sleeping patterns are not a setback at this stage; they are simply a stage — and they will pass.

Establish a quiet time for yourself so that you can recharge your batteries

Even if naptime is a thing of the past, you can still insist on some quiet time — and it's a very good idea. Children who are unable to sleep-in day-care settings still spend quiet time on their cots. If you implement the same strategy at home, you will receive a much-needed break and your child will develop the valuable skill of quietly entertaining himself.

To create a quiet period, choose an early afternoon time. If it does become a nap, it will have no effect on his nighttime sleep. Then take the following steps:

Prepare your child by informing him that he requires some alone time in his room to rest. He may protest that he is not tired, but inform him firmly and neutrally that it is time for him to go to his room. Take him there and tell him, "Have a good night's sleep — I'll see you soon."

This is a quiet period but not necessarily a sleepy period, so inform him that he is not required to be in his bed. Provide him with toys and books, or allow him to listen to a cassette. Expect him to remain awake, though you may later see him and Teddy zonked on the floor together.

If he refuses to remain in his room, use a gate to create a secure, escape-proof haven for him.

You can create a small ritual to indicate the end of quiet time. For instance, provide him with a digital clock so he can announce when time is up, or, even better, play a musical tape or CD that will play for as long as you want the quiet time to last. When the music stops, he knows it's time to take action once more. However, there will be no cheating: Choosing a three-hour Wagner opera is unjust!

When your child has a great deal of independence in his room, you must ensure that the environment is completely safe. Examine outlets, lamp cords, and toys with small parts that can be swallowed (or stuffed up his nose!).

Resolving Common Bedtime Issues

Apart from sleep issues, no toddler issue concerns parents more than potty training. Having your neighbor assure you that no one has ever walked down the aisle in diapers is little consolation when your child is on her twentieth pair of training pants and the preschool is refusing to admit Junior until he keeps his pee and poop to himself.

When you combine sleep deprivation and potty training, you have a recipe for high anxiety.

The lowdown on nighttime poop (and pee)

The two- to three-year-old stage is ideal for potty training. This new development complicates sleep routines, as you now have to figure out how to keep her clean and dry while everyone else is sleeping!

Parents frequently ask how to deal with pee and poop while still getting some sleep, and we address the top two in this section, offering tips for maintaining your sanity once the diaper days (and nights) are over.

When can I expect my child to sleep through the night?

Surprisingly, staying dry at night has nothing to do with daytime toilet use. And, while some children do this well before their parents begin potty training them, children cannot be taught to stay dry at night.

Indeed, children frequently follow in their mother's or father's footsteps. Therefore, to determine when your child will be ready to sleep through the night, inquire of your parents when you reached this milestone. Although the majority of children stop wetting the bed by their fifth birthday, those who do so later often have a relative who did as well; it's not as genetic as blue eyes, but there is a strong familial connection.

Indeed, when both parents were over the age of five prior to reaching the dry-at-night stage, their toddler has an 80% chance of doing the same.

Boys are more likely than girls to develop this ability later in life.

However, the majority of pediatricians do not consider it bedwetting until a child reaches the age of six. A child who wets the sheets is still within normal developmental limits up to that point.

It's beneficial to understand the difference between day and night as you work on toilet training. Dryness at night is primarily a physical issue; it occurs when your child's body is prepared. On the other hand, daytime dryness is a psychological as well as a physical process (a tug of war between infanthood and adulthood).

How do I know when my baby is ready to transition from nighttime diapers to daytime diapers?

Potty training can be a stressful time for parents, and many choose to keep their toddlers in diapers at night in order to create a haven of calm. However, diapers must eventually be discarded. You'll know if your child is ready to transition if:

She awakens with a completely dry (or nearly dry) diaper.

She is wet in the morning but appears to have urinated shortly before or shortly after waking up.

She is at least three years old and is requesting to sleep in her pantyhose.

Your intuition tells you that she may take an eternity to awaken and make her way to the bathroom, owing to the comfort and convenience of the diaper.

Even if your child is still soaked in the morning, as she approaches her third birthday, you may wish to discontinue diaper use.

Although large-size diapers are available, children this age frequently perceive diapers as baby items and would rather suffer through some wet sheets than continue wearing the white badge of infanthood.

How do I potty train my infant if he or she sleeps in a crib at night?

If your snookum's potty trains first, you'll need a plan for the night, as she won't be able to get out of the crib on her own. Depending on your individual sleep requirements, you can follow one of the following plans:

At night, use diapers.

Assist her when the urge to urinate strikes.

Fancy pants: Tales from the Crib

Violeta received three packages of lovely new undies from her aunt for her third birthday. Violeta insisted on wearing her new fancy pants to bed that night. Violeta had been using the restroom during the day for several months, but each morning she awoke swimming. Her mother, Sofia, was concerned that Violeta's soaking-wet new undies would affect her self-esteem the following morning.

However, Sofia caved in because it was Violeta's birthday and she was so insistent.

The following morning, she discovered Violeta drenched to the gills but unconcerned in the least. Violeta assisted her mother in stripping the bed's wet sheets, took a quick bath, changed into dry pantyhose, and was ready to face the day.

Sofia was relieved Violeta handled the experience so well, but she wasn't looking forward to daily laundry of wet sheets. Sofia layered three layers of absorbent towels over the bottom sheet each night to make life easier for both of them. Thus, the sheet beneath remained dry, and Violeta was able to remove the damp towels each morning. Violeta continued to wet the bed, but wearing her fancy pants and handling her own wet towels in the morning gave her a sense of maturity. Violeta's ability to care for her own wet clothing enabled her to be self-sufficient and eliminated the need for Sofia to intervene.

Violeta's father wet the bed until he was six, and Violeta followed suit.

However, she maintained control of her own body and stopped wetting the bed when she was physically capable — without intervention from Mom or Dad.

If your child frequently uses the "I have to go potty!" line but you believe it is a ruse to get you into the bedroom in the middle of the night, consider converting the room to a crib and restricting her movement out of the room with a gate.

If your child continues to request assistance with a midnight pee, you can leave a night light on and even place a small portable potty in the room to eliminate the need for your tot to leave her room.

What am I to do when

B.M. denotes blackmail?

A child who is potty trained or on the verge of becoming potty trained quickly learns that the words "I have to go to the bathroom" have an instant and almost magical effect on parents. What better way to entice Mommy or Daddy back into the nursery at night than to utter that evocative phrase? It's a rare parent who can say "No" to such a basic and necessary request. Maintain a loving but firm stance, however, and foster an environment in which your child can care for herself.

If your child sleeps in a bed instead of a crib, you can anticipate her using the bathroom independently — even at night. Parents who continue to think of their toddlers as infants frequently worry that this expectation is too high for a small child. However, toddlers find these steps quite simple, and they respond positively to the very adult feeling of self-care (although some resistance is expected at first).

If your child refuses to do potty chores on her own (and attempts to involve you) at night, she is requesting your attention, not your assistance. Take this opportunity to tell her, "You're becoming quite mature, and you're capable of doing this." You're likely to notice that she gains new confidence and becomes more willing to take on additional big girl tasks.

It may take a few nights to get the message across, but if you follow these steps, you will eventually succeed:

Keep a night light on in your toddler's room to assist her in locating the door.

Keep a small light on in your child's bathroom if it is connected to her bedroom.

If your toddler's room is down the hall from the bathroom, place a portable potty chair in his or her room. Place it on an old bathroom rug to aid in the absorption of any spills.

Put your toddler in pull-ups, training pants, or regular underwear to avoid her requiring your assistance in pulling her pants down.

Additionally, purchase pajamas with elastic waistbands that are easy to slip down (or consider dressing a girl in a nightgown).

Avoid one-piece flannel footies; they are simply too difficult for a toddler to manage.

Arrange a few pairs of clean undies and dry pajamas on the floor in case your child accidentally wets herself and requires a change.

Keep some dry towels on hand for your child to use if the sheets are wet.

Face-to-face with the bogeyman

Each month, your child increases his or her ability to communicate and understand others. Surprisingly, this heightened mental capacity does not always translate into more rational thought and behavior. On the contrary, children begin developing out-of-control fears of all kinds at the age of two. Two- to three-year-old confuse fantasy and reality because they lack the necessary life experience to discern the difference. If you're not convinced, take a group of 3-year-olds to a magician. Even the most incredible tricks will fail to impress them — after all, from their perspective, things that appear and disappear are a natural part of life! (For more information on how your child's thinking influences her behavior, see Section 7.)

Recognize the difficulty inherent in distinguishing between the real and the unreal

Your child's fears of bogeymen in the closet and monsters beneath the bed stem from an incomplete understanding of the world. As a result, the Teletubbies are as real to him as his next-door neighbors, and Oscar the Grouch may be a resident of your trash can. This conflation of the real person and the fictitious character can be perplexing and downright frightening. Therefore, if you are awakened by a crying toddler insisting, "There is a monster under my bed!" it is not a ploy to gain your attention. That monster, from his vantage point, is real.

While an infant is secure in the knowledge that his needs will be met and his discomforts will be alleviated, children between the ages of 2 and 3 become more aware of their own vulnerability and the fact that their parents are not truly all-powerful.

A fascinating illustration of this shift is that a toddler who falls and injures himself may yell at or even strike a parent who comes to console him. It's almost as if he's asking, "Why did you allow me to be injured?" On some level, he still expects you to protect him from everything, but when he realizes that you cannot, he is forced to deal with some pretty significant, complex emotions. As a result, you're likely to observe some unusual behavior along the way — some of it involving sleep.

Demonstration of their

falsity

Due to the darkness and his separation from you, your child's new fears and feelings may be amplified at night. If he summons you, the following tips will help make those things-that-go-bump-in-the-night a little less frightening:

Avoid mocking your child's concerns. Recognize them with your words and actions.

Verbally reassure your child. Assure him that you understand his fear of the monster, but that monsters do not exist.

Demonstrate to your child that he is safe. Prove it by using a broom or a flashlight to search all the scary hiding places.

Keep a small flashlight in the bedroom of your child. This way, he can inspect the room for himself while you are away.

(Ensure that the flashlight is suitable for toddlers — not too heavy, no sharp edges — and consider taping the battery lid shut to prevent small fingers from accessing the batteries.)

Install a nightlight in your child's room. Attempt to locate a location where it does not cast frightening shadows!

Maintain a tranquil and quiet bedtime ritual. Choose books that are free of frightening images or words. This is not the time for tales of snakes, spiders, or large, frightening dragons.

Of course, your child's fears are not limited to imaginary creatures. Several of them deal with all-too-real monsters such as robbers and murderers. If your small pumpkin is concerned about these genuine bad guys, reassure him that it is your responsibility to keep him safe and that you will do so.

Often, toddlers develop fears as a result of watching television or movies, so be extremely cautious about what your child learns from the big or small screen. Even G-rated films are not always safe, as what you consider to be tame or even cute may be frightening to a toddler. Choose toddler-friendly shows and movies, and try to view them through the eyes of a child to anticipate problems.

Simply because your toddler wants to watch a show repeatedly does not mean it is not frightening. Often, children are simply attempting to regain control over their fear. (Adults do this when they repeatedly recount a frightening experience.) Rather than allowing your child to continue watching an upsetting film or television show, speak with him about the frightening scenes and help him understand that they are made-up.

Inform him that you understand the film was too frightening and that you're putting it away. He may object initially, but he is relieved on the inside that you are shielding him from the frightening images.